Fast Facts

Fast Facts:
Schizophrenia

Third edition

D0773811

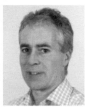

Shôn W Lewis BSc MD FRCPsych
Professor of Adult Psychiatry
University of Manchester
Manchester, UK

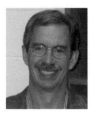

Robert W Buchanan MD
Professor of Psychiatry
Maryland Psychiatric Research Center
Department of Psychiatry
University of Maryland School of Medicine
Baltimore, Maryland, USA

Declaration of Independence
This book is as balanced and as practical as we can make it.
Ideas for improvement are always welcome:
feedback@fastfacts.com

HEALTH PRESS

Fast Facts: Schizophrenia
First published 1998; reprinted 2000
Second edition September 2002
Third edition February 2007

Health Press Limited, Elizabeth House, Queen Street, Abingdon,
Oxford OX14 3LN, UK
Tel: +44 (0)1235 523233
Fax: +44 (0)1235 523238

Book orders can be placed by telephone or via the website.
For regional distributors or to order via the website, please go to:
www.fastfacts.com
For telephone orders, please call 01752 202301 (UK), +44 1752 202301 (Europe),
1 800 247 6553 (USA, toll free) or +1 419 281 1802 (Americas).

Fast Facts is a trademark of Health Press Limited.

The publisher and the authors have made every effort to ensure the accuracy of this
book, but cannot accept responsibility for any errors or omissions.

For all drugs, please consult the product labeling approved in your country for
prescribing information.

A CIP record for this title is available from the British Library.

ISBN 978-1-903734-93-3

Lewis SW (Shôn)
Fast Facts: Schizophrenia/
Shôn W Lewis, Robert W Buchanan

Typesetting and page layout by Zed, Oxford, UK.
Printed by Fine Print (Services) Ltd, Oxford, UK.

Text printed with vegetable inks on fully biodegradable and
recyclable paper manufactured from sustainable forests.

Low emissions
during production

Low
chlorine

Sustainable
forests

Glossary of abbreviations

AMPA: α-amino-3-hydroxy-5-methyl-4-isoxazole propionic acid; a glutamatergic neurotransmitter

BOLD imaging: blood-oxygen-level-dependent imaging; magnetic resonance imaging that uses the natural paramagnetic properties of hemoglobin as it deoxygenates to produce an image of regional cerebral blood flow

CBT: cognitive-behavioral therapy

CPZE: chlorpromazine equivalent; the approximate dose equivalent to 100 mg of chlorpromazine (relative potency)

CSF: cerebrospinal fluid

CT: computed tomography

DTI: diffusion tensor imaging; a type of magnetic resonance imaging that allows visualization of white matter tracts

DUP: duration of untreated psychosis

DZ: dizygotic (of two fertilized eggs); dizygotic twins are non-identical

EPS: extrapyramidal side effects, e.g. akinesia, dystonia, akathisia and tremor

fMR: functional magnetic resonance; a means of imaging based on the same principles as BOLD imaging that can measure tiny metabolic changes in active areas of the brain

GPI: general paresis of the insane

MRI: magnetic resonance imaging

MZ: monozygotic (of one fertilized egg); monozygotic twins are identical

NMDA: N-methyl-D-aspartate

NMS: neuroleptic malignant syndrome; characterized by muscle rigidity, autonomic instability, fever and changes in mental status

PEG: pneumoencephalography; an old imaging technique based on the X-ray contrast of air injected into the lumbar subarachnoid space, bone and brain tissue

PET: positron emission tomography; a functional imaging technique used to measure glucose metabolism, regional cerebral blood flow or receptor occupancy

Potency: the quantity of a drug needed to have an effect

rCBF: regional cerebral blood flow

SPECT: single-photon emission computed tomography; functional imaging similar to, but less versatile than, PET

STG: superior temporal gyrus

TD: tardive dyskinesia; a major adverse effect associated with all conventional antipsychotics characterized by abnormal, involuntary movements; primarily affects the muscles of the tongue and face

VCFS: velocardiofacial syndrome; a genetic disorder characterized by palate and facial abnormalities, heart defects and various psychiatric symptoms

Introduction

Schizophrenia is a strange and often devastating disorder that starts in early life and can lead to lifelong disability. It is one of the major public health challenges.

Recent advances in research have given tantalizing insights as to the causes of schizophrenia, in particular the role of specific genes and psychosocial factors. How much do genes matter? Are psychological and social factors important? What about the effects of street drugs?

In this third edition of *Fast Facts: Schizophrenia* we cover what is new and promising in the understanding of risk factors, and cognitive and brain deficits. We also review new drug and non-drug treatment strategies, and consider the prospects these hold for better clinical and social outcomes.

1 A brief history

Preclassical and classical descriptions

The earliest descriptions of symptoms associated with the diagnosis of schizophrenia date back to preclassical cultures. Such symptoms were then considered to be the manifestations of supernatural forces invading the individual, often as punishment for immoral behavior.

In ancient Greece and Rome, the focus for studying and understanding mental illnesses moved towards a naturalistic standpoint. Early Greek physicians described delusions of grandeur, paranoia and deterioration in cognitive functions and personality. These behaviors were attributed generally to disturbances among the associations of the four bodily humors: blood, yellow bile, black bile and phlegm.

Medieval times

In medieval times, particularly in Western societies, there was a return to the preclassical moralistic or superstitious perspectives on psychotic behavior. The classical models of illness were largely kept alive by Arab physicians, who practiced medicine according to the ideas of Hippocrates, Aristotle and Galen. These classical conceptualizations of psychosis went unchanged until the Renaissance.

The Renaissance

In Western cultures, the Renaissance led to a reemergence of interest in classical thought, with a reawakening of the conceptualization of mental illnesses, including psychoses, as naturalistic disorders. The first European psychiatric hospitals were established during this period. The 17th and 18th centuries saw an explosion of information about the workings of the body, which led to a more rational and scientific approach to diseases and the study of the mind. Organic etiologies of mental illness were adopted, and the initial descriptions and classifications of these disorders were attempted.

19th century

In the first part of the 19th century, the foundations for the modern concept of schizophrenia were established (Table 1.1). An early diagnostic system emerged and various mental illnesses were described, including epilepsy, melancholia, mania and the dementing psychotic

TABLE 1.1

Major landmarks in the development of the concept of schizophrenia

Haslam J, 1809	Published a treatise on a type of insanity that occurs in the young
Esquirol JED, 1838	Described the prognosis and long-term course of different forms of insanity
Morel BA, 1860	Described 'démence précoce' (dementia praecox), a progressive deterioration evolving quickly in young persons
Kahlbaum KL, 1863	Described a form of insanity characterized by abnormal posturing: 'catatonia'
Hecker E, 1871	Described a form of insanity characterized by onset in puberty, evolution through successive affective states, ultimately resulting in states of psychological weakness and mental deficiency: 'hebephrenia'
Kraepelin E, 1898–9	Grouped together as a single illness dementia praecox and the formerly separate entities hebephrenia, catatonia and paranoid psychosis. Distinguished dementia praecox from manic–depressive illness on the basis of disease course and long-term outcome
Bleuler E, 1911	Recognized that patients with dementia praecox did not always deteriorate, coined the term schizophrenia and described fundamental symptoms
Kasanin J, 1933	Introduced the concept of schizoaffective disorder
Langfeldt G, 1939	Introduced the concept of schizophreniform disorder
Schneider K, 1946 (translated 1959)	Proposed the existence of pathognomonic, or first-rank, symptoms

disorders, which included schizophrenia and general paresis of the insane (GPI). However, a general approach that could integrate the diverse manifestations of mental illness into distinct clinical syndromes was lacking. The situation was complicated by the overlap in the clinical presentation of these disorders. Furthermore, the clinical presentation of an individual could change over time, and patients with the same symptoms could have different outcomes.

20th century

Two developments led to the eventual delineation of schizophrenia from the other dementing psychoses. First, the limitations of cross-sectional descriptions of symptoms for classifying mental disorders led to the emergence of a new system based on unified causes, clinicopathological correlations and the longitudinal course and prognosis of presumed disorders. The other development was the identification of the spirochete as the causal agent in GPI (Figure 1.1). In the 19th century, GPI was a common form of insanity. Its symptom manifestations were diverse and overlapped extensively with schizophrenic symptomatology. The identification of GPI as syphilitic

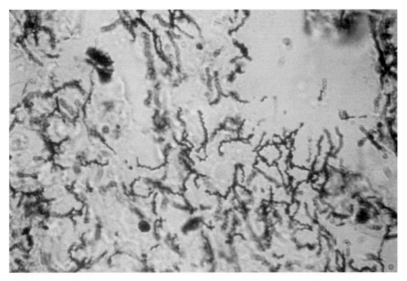

Figure 1.1 Micrograph showing spirochetes, identified as the agents causing a major 19th-century mental illness – general paresis of the insane.

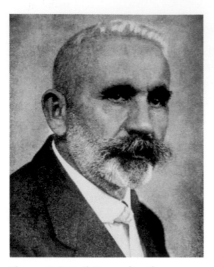

Figure 1.2 Emil Kraepelin, the German psychiatrist who identified dementia praecox (schizophrenia). His students included Alzheimer.

insanity helped Emil Kraepelin (Figure 1.2) to delineate the two other major patterns of insanity: manic–depressive psychosis and dementia praecox (or dementia of the young: schizophrenia), and to group together under the heading of dementia praecox the previously disparate categories of insanity, including hebephrenia, paranoia and catatonia.

In differentiating dementia praecox from manic–depressive disorder, Kraepelin emphasized the early onset and what he believed to be the inevitable deteriorating course of dementia praecox, compared with the relatively good outcome of manic–depressive illness. Kraepelin also described what he thought were the two main pathological processes in patients with schizophrenia:

'On the one hand we observe a weakening of those emotional activities which permanently form the mainsprings of volition ... mental activity and instinct for occupation become mute. The result of this part of the process is emotional dullness, failure of mental activities, loss of mastery over volition, of endeavor, and of ability for independent action. The essence of personality is thereby destroyed, the best and most precious part of its being, as Griesinger once expressed it, torn from her ...

The second group of disorders ... consists in the loss of the inner unity of the activities of intellect, emotion, and volition in themselves and among one another. Stransky speaks of an annihilation of the "intrapsychic coordination" ... this annihilation presents itself to us in the disorders of association described by Bleuler, in incoherence of the train of thought, in the sharp change of moods as well as in desultoriness and derailments in practical work ... the near connections between thinking and feeling, between deliberation and emotional activity on the one hand, and practical work on the other is more or less lost. Emotions do not correspond to ideas.' (*Dementia Praecox and Paraphrenia*, 1919).

The former process corresponds to our current concept of the negative symptoms, and the latter to the positive symptoms, of schizophrenia.

In 1911, Eugen Bleuler (Figure 1.3), recognizing that dementia was not a necessary characteristic of dementia praecox, suggested the term 'schizophrenia' (splitting of the mind) for the disorder. Bleuler believed that schizophrenia represented a syndrome consisting of several disorders that shared a common psychopathology. He also introduced the concept of primary and secondary schizophrenic symptoms; his four primary symptoms (the four 'A's) were:

- abnormal associations
- autistic behavior and thinking
- abnormal affect
- ambivalence.

Of these four symptoms, Bleuler viewed as central to the illness the loss of association between thought processes, and that between thought, emotion and behavior.

Since Kraepelin and Bleuler, there have been relatively few modifications of the description of schizophrenia. The diagnostic categories of schizophreniform and schizoaffective disorder were introduced in the 20th century, but these categories largely represent refinements in the boundary between schizophrenia and the affective disorders.

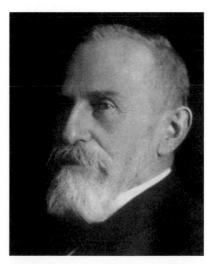

Figure 1.3 Eugen Bleuler, the Swiss psychiatrist who coined the term 'schizophrenia'. His students included Jung.

11

Current views

Currently, schizophrenia has the status of a syndrome resulting from multiple genetic and environmental causal pathways. These pathways produce disorders of normal brain function, which give rise to positive and negative symptoms, cognitive impairments and functional disabilities. These manifestations and their long-term course are used to differentiate schizophrenia from other forms of psychosis. However, recent neuroimaging and neuropsychological studies and molecular biology have paradoxically brought us back to the question that plagued Kraepelin and Bleuler: are schizophrenia and bipolar disorders separate diseases or do they represent ends of a continuum that includes schizoaffective disorder and unipolar depression?

Key points – a brief history

- Schizophrenia was first clearly identified in the 1890s.
- Its characteristic features were an early onset and a chronic course.
- Kraepelin described two characteristic psychopathological processes.
- Bleuler introduced the concept of primary and secondary symptoms.

Key references

Bleuler E. *Dementia Praecox or the Group of Schizophrenias* (1911). Translated by Zinken J. New York: International Universities Press, 1950.

Howells JG, ed. *The Concept of Schizophrenia: Historical Perspectives*. Washington, DC: American Psychiatric Press, 1991.

Kraepelin E. *Dementia Praecox and Paraphrenia* (1919). Translated by Barclay RM. Huntington, WV: Robert E Krieger, 1971.

Diagnostic criteria

Whether or not schizophrenia can be classified as a disease has been much debated. Strictly speaking, schizophrenia is a syndrome – a disorder for which there is no objective test or pathology, but which is identified by a characteristic cluster of symptoms that last for a certain time. In the 1930s, Kurt Schneider reviewed many case records and listed eight symptoms that he considered diagnostic of schizophrenia. These specific types of delusions and hallucinations became known as 'Schneider's first-rank symptoms' (Table 2.1), although they also occur occasionally in other serious psychiatric disorders.

TABLE 2.1

Schneider's first-rank symptoms of schizophrenia

Thought insertion, withdrawal or broadcasting	The experience of one's thoughts being put into or taken out of one's head, or broadcast to others. Collectively known as 'thought interference'
Passivity experiences	Experience that one's thoughts or actions are physically being controlled by an external force: 'made actions'
Delusional perception	A normal perception followed suddenly by a seemingly unrelated, fully formed delusion. Rare
Echo de la pensée	Hallucination of a voice repeating one's own thoughts
Running commentary	Hallucination describing one's current actions
Third-person auditory hallucinations	Voices describing patient as 'he' or 'she'

The loosening of the diagnostic boundaries in schizophrenia became a concern in the early 1970s. A series of studies showed that clinicians varied widely in their diagnosis of schizophrenia, which was made twice as often in North America than in Europe. As a result, operational diagnostic criteria, such as the Research Diagnostic Criteria of Endicott and Spitzer, were developed, initially for use in research, to try to standardize diagnosis. This approach gives a menu of possible symptoms and specifies that a certain number should be present for a minimum duration before a diagnosis can be made.

Since 1994, the two main classification systems in use worldwide have been the American Psychiatric Association's *Diagnostic and Statistical Manual of Mental Disorders*, Fourth Edition (DSM-IV, with a text revision in 2000: DSM-IV-TR) and the World Health Organization's *International Classification of Diseases*, Tenth Edition (ICD-10). The ICD-10 is mainly used outside North America. In their definitions of schizophrenia, the two systems are similar (Tables 2.2 and 2.3). Both diagnose schizophrenia with inter-rater reliabilities of at least 0.8, which compares well with those for many other medical disorders. Each specifies the presence of one first-rank-type symptom, or two symptoms from a list of positive and negative symptoms.

TABLE 2.2

DSM-IV diagnostic criteria for schizophrenia

A. Characteristic symptoms
Two (or more) of the following, each present for a substantial portion of time during a 1-month period (or less if successfully treated):
(1) delusions
(2) hallucinations
(3) disorganized speech (e.g. frequent derailment or incoherence)
(4) grossly disorganized or catatonic behavior
(5) negative symptoms (i.e. affective flattening, alogia or avolition)

Note: only one criterion A symptom is required if delusions are bizarre or hallucinations consist of a voice keeping up a running commentary on the person's behavior or thoughts, or two or more voices conversing with each other.   CONTINUED

TABLE 2.2 (CONTINUED)

B. Social/occupational dysfunction
For a substantial portion of the time since the onset of the disturbance, one or more major areas of functioning, such as work, interpersonal relations, or self-care, are markedly below the level achieved before the onset (or when the onset is in childhood or adolescence, failure to achieve expected level of interpersonal, academic or occupational achievement).

C. Duration
Continuous signs of the disturbance persist for at least 6 months. This 6-month period must include at least 1 month of symptoms (or less if successfully treated) that meet criterion A (i.e. active-phase symptoms) and may include periods of prodromal or residual symptoms. During these prodromal or residual periods, the signs of the disturbance may manifest as only negative symptoms or two or more symptoms listed in criterion A present in an attenuated form (e.g. odd beliefs, unusual perceptual experiences).

D. Schizoaffective and mood disorder exclusion
Schizoaffective disorder and mood disorder with psychotic features have been ruled out because either:
(1) no major depressive, manic or mixed episodes have occurred concurrently with the active-phase symptoms; or
(2) if mood episodes have occurred during active-phase symptoms, their total duration has been brief relative to the duration of the active and residual periods.

E. Substance/general medical condition exclusion
The disturbance is not due to the direct physiological effects of a substance (e.g. a drug of abuse, a medication) or a general medical condition.

F. Relationship to a pervasive development disorder
If there is a history of autistic disorder or another pervasive development disorder, the additional diagnosis of schizophrenia is made only if prominent delusions or hallucinations are also present for at least 1 month (or less if successfully treated).

TABLE 2.3

ICD-10 diagnostic criteria for schizophrenia

(a) Thought echo, thought insertion or withdrawal, or thought broadcasting

(b) Delusions of control, influence or passivity, clearly referred to body or limb movements or specific thoughts, actions or sensations; delusional perception

(c) Hallucinatory voices giving a running commentary on the patient's behavior, or discussing the patient among themselves, or other types of hallucinatory voices coming from some part of the body

(d) Persistent delusions of other kinds that are culturally inappropriate and completely impossible (e.g. being able to control the weather, or being in communication with aliens from another world)

(e) Persistent hallucinations in any modality, when accompanied either by fleeting or half-formed delusions without clear affective content, or by persistent over-valued ideas, or when occurring every day for weeks or months on end

(f) Breaks or interpolations in the train of thought, resulting in incoherence or irrelevant speech, or neologisms

(g) Catatonic behavior, such as excitement, posturing, or waxy flexibility, negativism, mutism and stupor

(h) 'Negative' symptoms, such as marked apathy, paucity of speech, and blunting or incongruity of emotional responses; it must be clear that these are not due to depression or to neuroleptic medication

Diagnostic guidelines

The normal requirement for a diagnosis of schizophrenia is a minimum of one clear symptom (usually two or more if less clearcut) belonging to any one of the groups (a) to (d), or symptoms from at least two of the groups (e) to (h); symptoms should have been clearly present for most of the time for 1 month or more.

Adapted from *The ICD-10 Classification of Mental and Behavioural Disorders. Diagnostic Criteria for Research*. Geneva: World Health Organization, 1993.

ICD-10, *International Statistical Classification of Diseases and Related Health Problems*, Tenth Edition.

The main differences are that the DSM-IV states a minimum duration of symptoms, including prodromal symptoms, of 6 months, and includes deterioration of social functioning, whereas the ICD-10 specifies just 1 month of symptoms. A classification of an acute form of schizophrenia in the ICD-10 is equivalent to a classification of schizophreniform disorder in the DSM-IV.

These differences mean that DSM-IV schizophrenia has a lower incidence and prevalence than ICD-10 schizophrenia, and has a worse prognosis as a result of the degree of chronicity in its definition. As there is a slight tendency for schizophrenia to be more chronic in men, the sex ratio shows a male predominance for DSM-IV schizophrenia that is less apparent by ICD-10 criteria.

Core symptoms

A large number of studies have found that the symptoms of schizophrenia usually segregate into three semi-independent symptom complexes (Table 2.4). The three-syndrome model was first proposed in the 1980s and has been confirmed in multiple subsequent studies.

The presence and severity of negative symptoms are more critical to the prognosis than hallucinations and delusions; negative symptoms

TABLE 2.4

The three-syndrome model of schizophrenia*

Syndrome	Symptom pattern
Hallucinations and delusions	Hallucinations Delusions
Negative symptoms	Alogia Affective flattening Avolition Anhedonia
Behavioral disorganization	Positive formal thought disorder Inappropriate affect Bizarre behavior

*Based on Buchanan and Carpenter, 1994.

include alogia (reduced amount of spontaneous speech), affective flattening, avolition (reduced willpower) and anhedonia (loss of the ability to experience pleasure). Negative symptoms can become progressively more severe, and often persist to some degree even when positive symptoms have improved.

It is important to distinguish between primary and enduring negative symptoms or deficit symptoms, which are indisputably part of the illness, and secondary negative symptoms. The latter can be similar in quality but result from a superimposed anxious or depressed mood, an impoverished, understimulating environment or the adverse effects of antipsychotic medication.

The third symptom complex – behavioral disorganization – refers to a disruption in the associations among affect, thought and behavior. Inappropriate affect is the loss of connection between affect and thought (e.g. the patient who laughs while talking about the death of a loved one). Positive formal thought disorder involves a disruption of the normal grammatical and syntactic use of conversational language, such that statements become connected in unusual ways ('knight's-move thinking'), words are used idiosyncratically (paraphasia) or are invented (neologisms), or speech is rambling with little information content (poverty of speech content). Bizarre behavior refers to the socially inappropriate or disorganized behavior frequently exhibited by patients with schizophrenia.

In addition to these three symptom complexes, patients with schizophrenia may also present with affective symptoms, including symptoms of anxiety, depression and mania.

Rating scales

The use of structured rating scales to assess symptoms and function allows us to track clinical change over time and to assess outcome. It is an increasingly important function in service and treatment evaluation.

Outcome of schizophrenia can be measured in terms of severity of symptoms, cognitive function or social outcome, or by related constructs such as quality of life or patient satisfaction (Table 2.5). The characteristics to look for in a rating scale are listed in Table 2.6.

TABLE 2.5

Measurable dimensions of outcome and rating scales

Outcome	Scale
Symptoms	Brief Psychiatric Rating Scale (BPRS)[1]
	Scales for the Assessment of Positive/
	Negative Symptoms (SAPS/SANS)[2]
	Positive and Negative Syndrome Scale
	(PANSS)[3]
	Calgary Depression Scale (CDS)[4]
Social functioning/	Social Functioning Scale (SFS)[5]
behavior/adjustment	Social Behavior Schedule (SBS)[6]
Global functioning	Global Assessment of Functioning (in DSM-IV)[7]
Quality of life	Quality of Life Interview (QOLI)[8]
	Quality of Life Scale (QLS)[9]
Cognitive function/	UCSD Performance-Based Skills
capacity	Assessment (UPSA)[10]
	Schizophrenia Cognition Rating Scale
	(SCoRS)[11]
Satisfaction with services	General Satisfaction Questionnaire[12]
Use of services	Hospital inpatient days
Occupational	Days in work

[1]Overall and Gorham 1961; [2]Andreasen et al.1992; [3]Kay et al. 1987;
[4]Addington et al. 1993; [5]Birchwood et al. 1990; [6]Wykes and Sturt 1986;
[7]Jones et al. 1995; [8]Lehman 1988; [9]Heinrichs et al. 1984; [10]Patterson et al. 2001;
[11]Keefe et al. 2006; [12]Huxley 1990.

TABLE 2.6

What are the characteristics to look for in a rating scale?

- Logical and understandable
- Relevant to the study population
- Proven validity (measures what it claims to measure)
- Proven reliability, between raters and over time
- Sensitivity to change
- Availability of training and manuals/video

Measurable dimensions of outcome and the most widely used rating scales used to make these assessments are detailed below.

Symptoms. The Positive and Negative Syndrome Scale (PANSS) is now the most widely used of the symptom rating scales. It comprises three subscales that rate positive, negative and general symptoms, respectively. It takes about 20 minutes to administer. Symptomatic patients score typically between 60 and 120, and a score reduction of 20% is clinically useful. Alternatively, the Brief Psychiatric Rating Scale (BPRS) and Scales for the Assessment of Positive/Negative Symptoms (SAPS/SANS) may be used to track changes in positive, negative and general symptoms. The Calgary Depression Scale (CDS) is designed specifically to assess depressive symptoms in patients with schizophrenia. The CDS has been shown to be reliable and to have good construct validity.

Social functioning is a less frequently measured, but very important, outcome. The Social Behavior Schedule (SBS) is probably the best instrument, although the administration of the instrument requires a caregiver.

Global functioning can be estimated very simply using the Global Assessment of Functioning (GAF). Based on anchor points, this gives a single score from 0 to 100 depending on how the person is functioning in general.

Quality of life is an increasingly important concept, but the best way of measuring it is controversial. The Quality of Life Scale (QLS) is probably the most widely used schizophrenia-specific scale. The QLS assesses four areas: interpersonal relations, instrumental role function, intrapsychic foundations, and common objects and activities. The Quality of Life Interview (QOLI) has also been extensively used to assess the quality of life of patients with schizophrenia. The QOLI is a structured interview designed to assess general life satisfaction and objective and subjective quality of life in the following life areas: living situation, family relations, social relations, daily activities, finances, safety and legal problems, work and school, and health.

Cognitive function/capacity. The assessment of cognitive function and capacity has become increasingly important with the increased recognition of the role that cognitive impairments play in poor outcome. The Schizophrenia Cognition Rating Scale (SCoRS) is an interview-based assessment of cognitive function. The UCSD Performance-Based Skills Assessment (UPSA) is a performance-based assessment of cognitive capacity, in which patients are asked to perform standardized role-play situations.

Key points – symptoms and diagnosis

- The *Diagnostic and Statistical Manual of Mental Disorders,* Fourth Edition (DSM-IV) and the *International Classification of Diseases,* Tenth Edition (ICD-10) provide the two principal diagnostic systems used to diagnose patients with schizophrenia.
- There are three major symptom clusters: hallucinations and delusions, negative symptoms and behavioral disorganization.
- Cognitive impairments and negative symptoms have the greatest prognostic importance for functional outcome.
- It is important to rate cognitive, social and behavioral outcomes, as well as symptoms.

Key references

Addington D, Addington J, Maticka-Tyndale E. Assessing depression in schizophrenia: the Calgary Depression Scale. *Br J Psychiatry Suppl* 1993;22:39–44.

American Psychiatric Association. *Diagnostic and Statistical Manual of Mental Disorders*, 4th edn (DSM-IV). Washington, DC: American Psychiatric Press, 1994.

Andreasen NC, Flaum M, Arndt S. The Comprehensive Assessment of Symptoms and History (CASH). An instrument for assessing diagnosis and psychopathology. *Arch Gen Psychiatry* 1992;49:615–23.

Birchwood M, Smith J, Cochrane R et al. The Social Functioning Scale. The development and validation of a new scale of social adjustment for use in family intervention programmes with schizophrenic patients. *Br J Psychiatry* 1990;157:853–9.

Buchanan RW, Carpenter WT. Domains of psychopathology: an approach to the reduction of heterogeneity in schizophrenia. *J Nerv Ment Dis* 1994;182:193–204.

Crow TJ. Positive and negative schizophrenic symptoms and the role of dopamine. *Br J Psychiatry* 1980;137:383–6.

Heinrichs DW, Hanlon TE, Carpenter WT Jr. The Quality of Life Scale: an instrument for rating the schizophrenic deficit syndrome. *Schizophr Bull* 1984;10:388–98.

Huxley PJ. The General Satisfaction Questionnaire (GSQ), Field Trial Results I: GSQ subscales. Manchester, UK: University of Manchester, Mental Health Social Work Research Unit, 1990.

Jones SH, Thornicroft G, Coffey M, Dunn G. A brief mental health outcome scale: reliability and validity of the Global Assessment of Functioning (GAF). *Br J Psychiatry* 1995;166:654–9.

Kay SR, Fishbein A, Opler LA. The positive and negative syndrome scale (PANSS) for schizophrenia. *Schizophr Bull* 1987;13:261–76.

Keefe RS, Poe M, Walker TM et al. The Schizophrenia Cognition Rating Scale: an interview-based assessment and its relationship to cognition, real-world functioning, and functional capacity. *Am J Psychiatry* 2006;163:426–32.

Kendell RE, Cooper JE, Gourlay AG et al. Diagnostic criteria of American and British psychiatrists. *Arch Gen Psychiatry* 1971;25:123–30.

Kirkpatrick B, Buchanan RW, Ross DE, Carpenter WT Jr. A separate disease within the syndrome of schizophrenia. *Arch Gen Psychiatry* 2001;58:165–71.

Lehman AF. A quality of life interview for the chronically mentally ill. *Eval Program Planning* 1988;11:51–62.

Liddle PF. The symptoms of chronic schizophrenia. A re-examination of the positive–negative dichotomy. *Br J Psychiatry* 1987;151:145–51.

Overall JE, Gorham DE. The Brief Psychiatric Rating Scale. *Psychol Rep* 1961;10:799–812.

Patterson TL, Goldman S, McKibbin CL et al. UCSD Performance-Based Skills Assessment: development of a new measure of everyday functioning for severely mentally ill adults. *Schizophr Bull* 2001;27:235–45.

World Health Organization. *The ICD-10 Classification of Mental & Behavioural Disorders. Diagnostic Criteria for Research*. Geneva: World Health Organization, 1993.

Wykes T, Sturt E. The measurement of social behaviour in psychiatric patients: an assessment of the reliability and validity of the SBS schedule. *Br J Psychiatry* 1986;148:1–11.

Knowledge of how schizophrenia is distributed within and between cultures is an important clue to possible theories of causation, as well as important in planning mental health services. The development of agreed, reliable definitions of the diagnosis has been crucial to epidemiological research. Since the late 1990s, how we think about the geographic distribution of schizophrenia has changed. The current state of knowledge is described here.

How common?

The incidence of schizophrenia is the number of new cases appearing, expressed either annually or as lifetime risk. The prevalence of schizophrenia is the number of cases at any one time point. These figures depend on whether the *International Classification of Diseases*, Tenth Edition (ICD-10) or the *Diagnostic and Statistical Manual of Mental Disorders*, Fourth Edition (DSM-IV; or the previous, similar DSM-III-R) criteria are used. Because of the 6-month, rather than 1-month, criterion in the DSM (see pages 14–17), the incidence and prevalence will be lower with DSM-IV criteria than with those of ICD-10. Large, community-based surveys of geographically defined areas yield prevalence estimates of between 0.2% and 0.7%. Incidence studies of epidemiological samples show that there will be about 2 new cases of ICD schizophrenia, or about 1 new case of DSM schizophrenia, per 10 000 population each year.

How global?

Schizophrenia exists in all cultures in all countries. The symptoms are surprisingly similar around the globe. Using clinical raters reliably trained to use the same diagnostic criteria, the World Health Organization showed, in two large field studies in 12 centers in ten developed and developing countries, that narrowly defined schizophrenia had a similar incidence in all countries. However, there are several important differences. Although narrowly defined schizophrenia was recorded at roughly similar rates, broadly defined schizophrenia was found to differ in prevalence between countries. Furthermore, the outcome of the illness was substantially better in developing than in developed countries. Why this should be is unknown. Possible explanations include different combinations of etiologic factors, or differences in factors known to aid recovery, such as family support or decreased environmental stimulation.

Age, sex and season of birth

The incidence of schizophrenia is slightly more common in men. Men are also more likely than women to develop enduring negative symptoms. The peak age of onset in men is from 21 to 26 years, whereas in women it is from 25 to 32 years (Figure 3.1).

A well-replicated finding is that, compared with the general population, people who go on to develop schizophrenia are about 8% more likely to have been born in late winter or early spring (January to March in the northern hemisphere; July to September in the southern hemisphere). The reasons for this phenomenon are still not clear. Suggestions that this is due to a seasonal pattern of intrauterine infection would correlate better with an increase in summer births, since the main

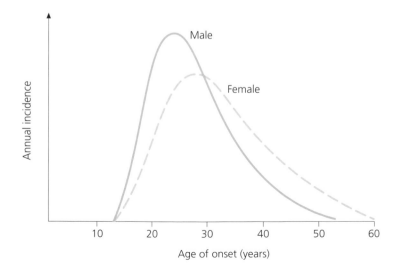

Figure 3.1 Annual incidence of schizophrenia by sex.

impact would be during the first trimester. An alternative explanation is an alteration in the normal seasonal pattern of conceptions (slightly higher in summer) in parents carrying a schizophrenia gene.

Migration and ethnicity

It has been recognized since the 1990s that ethnic minority groups have increased rates of psychosis. In the UK, rates of schizophrenia and bipolar disorder are higher in several ethnic groups, particularly black people from the Caribbean, a finding also reported in other European countries. This is not an artifact of misdiagnosis, as claimed originally, but is probably linked to aversive psychosocial experiences. The size of the effect has been shown to depend on the cultural milieu, with rates highest for Caribbean black people living in mainly white areas.

City life and schizophrenia

It has long been known that rates of schizophrenia are higher in urban than in rural areas. Early surveys seemed to show that this was due to the drift of people into urban areas after the illness started, rather than to higher rates of new cases in cities. However, recent large studies have confirmed that new cases arise more commonly in cities, with the rates being proportional to the degree of urbanization. This appears to be an unexpectedly large effect. The relative risk for large-city dwellers compared with that for rural residents is only two- to threefold (see Table 5.2, page 38) but, because much of the population lives in cities, the proportion of schizophrenia that can be explained on the basis of this factor is about one-third. Being brought up in a city appears to be the critical factor, and the risk increases the more childhood years spent in an urban environment. The factors associated with city life that lead to this higher incidence remain to be clarified. The data suggest that those with a genetic vulnerability are most at risk of the effects of urban upbringing.

Course and outcome

The best outcome studies are those that prospectively follow a cohort of consecutive first-episode patients, ideally from a defined geographic area, for at least 5 years. However, such studies are rare. Summarizing

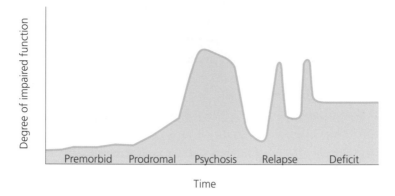

Figure 3.2 Profile of typical life course in schizophrenia.

the best long-term studies available, there is a consensus that 15–20% of patients will make a complete recovery without relapse. At the other extreme, about 15% will effectively never recover from their first episode, remaining symptomatic and needing long-term, high levels of social and medical input. Between these two poles, most patients will recover at least partly from their first episode, but will not return to their premorbid level of functioning, or will suffer future relapses, or both (Figure 3.2). In total, 5% of patients commit suicide, but it is difficult to predict occurrence. Young men in the first 3 years of their illness are most at risk.

Clues to long-term outcome can be gleaned from demographic factors and from the pattern of the first episode. Robust predictors of outcome are summarized in Table 3.1.

Community psychotic symptoms

Recent surveys have shown that unexpectedly high rates of apparently healthy people in the community, perhaps 5–15%, report isolated psychosis-like symptoms, such as hearing a voice, from time to time. Such symptoms do not distress them and do not cause them to seek help. One school of thought is that this represents part of the phenotype of schizophrenia or at least psychosis (Figure 3.3), and that a proportion of these individuals may progress to having 'prodromal' symptoms, described in Chapter 11 (page 93), of whom a proportion will develop schizophrenia.

TABLE 3.1

Well-established predictors of outcome

Factor	Good outcome	Poor outcome
Demographic	• Female • Married	• Male • Single
Genetic	• Family history of mood disorder	• Family history of schizophrenia
Onset	• Good premorbid adjustment • Acute onset • Life event at onset • Prompt treatment	• Schizoid traits • Slow onset • Long duration of untreated psychosis • Onset under 17 years old
Symptoms	• Affective symptoms	• Negative symptoms • Obsessions • Bizarre delusions • Poor insight
Psychosocial	• Good response to treatment	• High expressed emotion • Substance misuse • Poor adherence to treatment

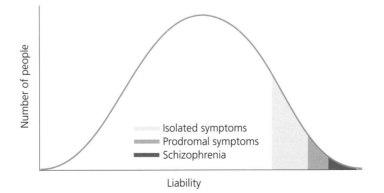

Figure 3.3 Liability-threshold model of schizophrenia. Everyone has a certain level of underlying liability – the sum of small risk factors – distributed normally in the population. Schizophrenia emerges above an extreme threshold. Lower thresholds probably exist for prodromal and isolated symptom states.

27

Key points – epidemiology

- The incidence of new cases of schizophrenia is 1–2 per 10 000 population per year.
- The condition exists in all countries and cultures, but prevalence rates vary.
- Onset is usually in early adult life; 20% will recover completely.
- Urban environments in childhood appear unexpectedly important in causing schizophrenia.

Key references

Harrison G, Croudace T, Mason P et al. Predicting the long-term outcome of schizophrenia. *Psychol Med* 1996;26:697–705.

Hopper K, Wanderling J. Revisiting the developed versus developing country distinction in course and outcome in schizophrenia: results from ISoS, the WHO collaborative followup project. International Study of Schizophrenia. *Schizophr Bull* 2000;26:835–46.

Kendler KS, Gallagher TJ, Abelson JM, Kessler RC. Lifetime prevalence, demographic risk factors and diagnostic validity of nonaffective psychosis assessed in a US community sample. The National Comorbidity Survey. *Arch Gen Psychiatry* 1996;53:1022–31.

Kirkbride JB, Fearon P, Morgan C et al. Heterogeneity in incidence rates of schizophrenia and other psychotic syndromes: findings from the 3-center AeSOP study. *Arch Gen Psychiatry* 2006;63:250–8.

McGrath J, Saha S, Welham J et al. A systematic review of the incidence of schizophrenia: the distribution of rates and the influence of sex, urbanicity, migrant status and methodology. *BMC Med* 2004;2:13.

Mortensen PB, Pedersen CB, Westergaard T et al. Effects of family history and place and season of birth on the risk of schizophrenia. *N Engl J Med* 1999;340:603–8.

Pedersen CB, Mortensen PB. Evidence of a dose–response relationship between urbanicity during upbringing and schizophrenia risk. *Arch Gen Psychiatry* 2001;58:1039–46.

Sartorius N, Jablensky A, Korten A et al. Early manifestations and first-contact incidence of schizophrenia in different cultures. A preliminary report on the initial evaluation phase of the WHO Collaborative Study on determinants of outcome of severe mental disorders. *Psychol Med* 1986;16:909–28.

The biggest single clue we have about the cause of schizophrenia is that it often runs in families. Although this observation was made first in the opening years of the 20th century, until relatively recently it was disputed whether or not this family clustering was truly a genetic effect.

Classic studies

The most straightforward studies in population genetics are family studies. Usually, a series of schizophrenic individuals, known as probands or index cases, is selected and rates of schizophrenia are assessed in their biological families. These rates are compared with rates in the families of control probands, usually healthy volunteers. To express the results as rates, the number of affected relatives is divided by the total number and is age-corrected for relatives who either are too young to have the disorder or are not yet through the age range at highest risk.

The risk of schizophrenia in relatives depends first on how close the relative is to the proband (Figure 4.1). Spouses are at slightly increased risk because of assortative mating (i.e. selection of similar partners). The diagnostic system used affects the risk to relatives, as it does prevalence, and fewer relatives will be diagnosed with DSM-IV schizophrenia than with ICD-10 schizophrenia. Recent studies have shown an unexpected effect of sex. Relatives of female probands have higher rates of schizophrenia than relatives of male probands.

Family studies can never give conclusive proof of genetic effects, as familiality could be due to a shared environmental factor. Nevertheless, family studies have shown that if there is a genetic effect, it does not follow a recognized Mendelian pattern of autosomal dominance, such as in Huntington's disease, or recessiveness, such as in cystic fibrosis.

Studies in twins and adopted children

Studies in twins involve probands with schizophrenia who are either identical (monozygotic: MZ) or non-identical (dizygotic: DZ). Concordance rates in the two types of twins are compared by looking

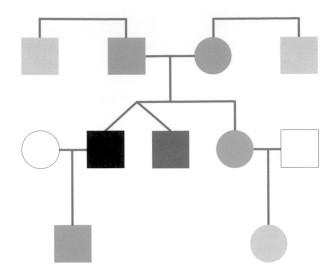

Figure 4.1 A genogram showing risk of schizophrenia in relatives. Proband (black); an identical twin (red) shares 100% of genes, risk 45%; a first-degree relative (blue) shares 50% of genes, risk 10%; a second-degree relative (yellow) shares 25% of genes, risk 3%.

at the rate at which co-twins also have schizophrenia. MZ twins share 100% of their genes and DZ twins share about 50%. The consensus from population-based studies is that concordance rates are about 45% for MZ co-twins compared with 15% for DZ co-twins. The fact that concordance is less than 100% in MZ twins suggests that non-genetic, environmental factors are also involved. However, the offspring of the unaffected MZ co-twins in discordant pairs also appear to be at increased risk of schizophrenia, suggesting that the co-twins still carry a genetic predisposition for the disease.

Adoption studies offer the most watertight evidence for genetic effects, as family environment is taken out of the equation. There are two types of study: follow-up and follow-back. Both methods have shown that it is biological parentage rather than adoptive parentage that predisposes to schizophrenia.

Follow-up studies trace the biological children of schizophrenic mothers, who were adopted into normal families at birth, and compare the number of offspring who develop schizophrenia with control adoptees of healthy mothers.

Follow-back studies start with a group of schizophrenic adults who were known to be adopted at birth. The biological parents are traced and their rates of illness compared with those in the biological parents of control adoptees.

The extended phenotype

The results from family, twin and adoption studies subjected to modern diagnostic criteria support the notion that a proportion of biological relatives of schizophrenic probands, while not having frank schizophrenia, have an unusual cluster of traits. This was previously called latent schizophrenia, but is now termed schizotypal personality disorder. A number of other schizophrenia spectrum disorders are found in the families of schizophrenic probands (Table 4.1).

Measurements of cognitive abnormalities provide an alternative approach for defining the phenotype. Impairments in attention, evoked potentials such as the P50 wave, working memory, and smooth-pursuit and saccadic eye movements are often seen in patients and their families. These cognitive abnormalities may be more sensitive than diagnostic categories for indicating the presence of genes for schizophrenia. They can supplement the use of diagnostic categories in genetic studies, enhancing the likelihood of detecting these genes.

TABLE 4.1

Disorders found at increased rates in families of schizophrenic probands

- Schizophrenia
- Schizoaffective disorder
- Delusional disorder
- Schizotypal disorder
- Atypical psychosis
- Major depression
- Bipolar disorder

What is the pattern of inheritance?

It is clear that schizophrenia is not transmitted in a Mendelian fashion. It conforms to the pattern of other 'complex' disorders, such as ischemic heart disease. Any model, however, must explain why schizophrenia is so common, with a lifetime prevalence approaching 1% (i.e. 20 times more common than the most common Mendelian disorder, cystic fibrosis). It must also explain why schizophrenia persists in the population when it is accompanied by obvious biological disadvantage.

The genome

Clinically, schizophrenia varies widely in its symptoms and course. This has often been taken as evidence for etiologic heterogeneity, either with several different mutations yielding slightly different clinical pictures, or with familial and non-familial forms. However, several mechanisms that may alter the extent to which a gene is expressed are known. Partial penetrance or variable expressivity can occur so that the same gene can produce a range of effects, such as in neurofibromatosis where the gene that produces an 'elephant man' effect in one person produces only a few skin speckles in another. Interaction between genes (epistasis) also occurs.

The size and power of studies performed indicates that there is unlikely to be any single gene that confers a relative risk of schizophrenia greater than threefold. Quantitative genetic studies have ruled out the explanation that it is a collection of single-gene disorders. The current picture is of a polygenic disorder with environmental factors acting on the penetrance of several susceptibility genes.

The search for genes in schizophrenia is difficult for several reasons (Table 4.2). The approach known as linkage analysis focuses either on multiply affected pedigrees apparently involving major genes, or on analysis of large samples of sibling pairs discordant for the disorder – so-called association studies. The second approach is better for genes of small effect and where the mode of inheritance is unclear. Either the search can be focused on so-called candidate genes, such as those coding for dopamine or glutamate receptors, or else a genome-wide search can be done where known genetic markers throughout the genome (polymorphisms) are used to locate the faulty gene, a technique known as positional cloning.

TABLE 4.2

Difficulties in the search for a gene in schizophrenia

- The limits of the phenotype are not well understood (e.g. should schizotypes be included?)
- The mode of inheritance is unclear; this is important for linkage analysis, but less so for association studies
- It is unclear which genes or chromosomes are candidates for linkage
- It is not known whether the results from studies of highly familial schizophrenia are applicable to all schizophrenia
- Genes probably have small individual effect, so large samples are needed

For 15 years, the search for linkage was disappointing, partly because sample sizes were too small. Recent advances in genome analysis have made the task of positional cloning much more efficient and statistically sensitive. Notable linkage has been confirmed in meta-analyses to regions on chromosomes 1q, 6p, 8p, 13q, 18p and 22q, supporting the notion that there are several susceptibility genes.

Of these, the evidence is strongest for the genes neuregulin (*NRG1*; 8p12), dysbindin (*DTNBP1*; 6p22) and *DISC1* (1q42) (Table 4.3). The *DISC1* linkage followed from the finding of a Scottish pedigree with a balanced 1;11 chromosomal translocation. The catechol-O-methyltransferase (*COMT*) gene is central to dopamine metabolism and has been studied because its location is close to the 22q11 region. The rare, neurodevelopmental velocardiofacial syndrome (VCFS) results from a gene deletion at 22q11, and schizophrenia develops in 25% of VCFS patients. A missense mutation in the *COMT* gene gives a valine-to-methionine substitution at codon 158, which produces an unstable enzyme, with reduced breakdown of dopamine. Individuals with this polymorphism have altered activity of the prefrontal cortex during working memory tasks. COMT inhibitors improve memory. The COMT genotype has also been shown to predict the degree of improvement in working memory and negative symptoms in schizophrenia treated with olanzapine.

TABLE 4.3

Susceptibility genes for schizophrenia

Gene	Evidence
NRG1	First identified in an Icelandic sample in 2002; encodes for proteins with a range of synaptogenesis and myelination functions
DTNBP1	First identified in an Irish sample in 2002; may act on presynaptic glutamate function
DISC1	Followed from the finding of a Scottish pedigree with balanced 1;11 chromosomal translocation; likely action on neuronal migration and intracellular transport
G30/DAO, G72/DAOA	First identified in a Russian sample in 2002; interacting pair of genes; DAO activates NMDA glutamate receptor
COMT	Slightly weaker evidence for linkage; established link between higher-activity valine allele at codon 158 and reduced frontal task performance in normal subjects
RGS4, GRM3	Weaker evidence

COMT, catechol-O-methyltransferase; DAO, D-amino acid oxidase;
DAOA, DAO activator; DISC1, disrupted-in-schizophrenia 1; DTNBP1, dysbindin;
NMDA, N-methyl-D-aspartate; NRG1, neuregulin.

The overlap with bipolar disorder

As genes predisposing to schizophrenia are now being discovered, there is renewed interest in the true association between schizophrenia and bipolar disorder. It has long been known that neither disorder 'breeds true'. The children of schizophrenic mothers have a sixfold increased risk of bipolar disorder, as well as higher rates of schizophrenia. Estimates suggest that perhaps 60% of the genetic variance for the two disorders is shared. Some genes, such as DISC1 and NRG1, appear to predispose to both disorders and perhaps have their strongest effect in schizoaffective disorders.

What particularly appear to characterize schizophrenia are the neurodevelopmental risk factors, such as delayed milestones and obstetric complications, which are not found in individuals who later develop bipolar disorder.

Key points – genetics

- Having a close relative with schizophrenia increases one's own risk 15-fold.
- Identical twins show a 45% concordance rate.
- Individual vulnerability genes exist.
- Genes are each of small effect and act additively.
- So far, 4–6 susceptibility genes have been identified, some of which also predispose to bipolar disorder.
- There are likely to be 15–20 genes in all.

Key references

Badner JA, Gershon ES. Meta-analysis of whole-genome linkage scans of bipolar disorder and schizophrenia. *Mol Psychiatry* 2002;7:405–11.

Cardno AG, Marshall EJ, MacDonald AM et al. Heritability estimates for psychotic disorders: the Maudsley twin psychosis study. *Arch Gen Psychiatry* 1999;56:162–8.

Chumakov I, Blumenfeld M, Guerassimenko O et al. Genetic and physiological data implicating the new human gene G72 and the gene for D-amino acid oxidase in schizophrenia. *Proc Natl Acad Sci USA* 2002;99:13675–80.

Craddock N, O'Donovan MC, Owen MJ. The genetics of schizophrenia and bipolar disorder: dissecting psychosis. *J Med Genet* 2005;42:193–204.

Kendler KS, Gruenberg AM. An independent analysis of the Danish Adoption Study of Schizophrenia. VI. The relationship between psychiatric disorders as defined by DSM-III in the relatives and adoptees. *Arch Gen Psychiatry* 1984;41:555–64.

Lewis CM, Levinson DF, Wise LH et al. Genome scan meta-analysis of schizophrenia and bipolar disorder, part II: schizophrenia. *Am J Hum Genet* 2003;73:34–48.

Stefansson H, Sigurdsson E, Steinthorsdottir V et al. Neuregulin 1 and susceptibility to schizophrenia. *Am J Hum Genet* 2002;71:877–92.

Straub RE, Jiang Y, MacLean CJ et al. Genetic variation in the 6p22.3 gene *DTNBP1*, the human ortholog of the mouse dysbindin gene, is associated with schizophrenia. *Am J Hum Genet* 2002;71:337–48.

5 Developmental theories and environmental factors

There has been a long dispute about whether schizophrenia is a degenerative brain disorder, as originally thought by Kraepelin, or whether it is better viewed as non-progressive.

During the 1990s, much attention was given to the 'neuro-developmental hypothesis' of schizophrenia. On the basis of the range of observations outlined in Table 5.1, it was suggested that a static lesion, either genetic or environmental in origin during brain development, expressed its effects as a function of the maturational stage of the brain. In the case of schizophrenia, the characteristic symptoms emerge only during the final stages of brain development in adolescence, at the stage when normal 'pruning' or elimination of excess synapses takes place.

Neurodevelopmental risk factors

Non-genetic factors probably account for about 30% of the risk for schizophrenia. Some established risk factors act early in life (Table 5.2).

TABLE 5.1

Evidence for schizophrenia being a neurodevelopmental disorder

- Association with obstetric complications, leading to earlier age of onset
- Unusual developmental trajectory in childhood, with cognitive and behavioral impairments
- Increased rate of minor physical anomalies
- Histological and morphological abnormalities at postmortem examination
- Association with known neurodevelopmental genetic disorders (e.g. velocardiofacial syndrome)

TABLE 5.2

Known early environmental risk factors for schizophrenia

Risk factor	Probable increase in risk
Intrauterine infections	1.2
Unwanted pregnancy	4
Rhesus compatibility	2
Birth complications	4
Winter birth	1.1
Childhood head injury	1.2
Childhood encephalitis	7
Adolescent cannabis use	3
Urban childhood	2.4
Ethnic minority status	2–6

Obstetric complications generally appear to increase the risk of schizophrenia. During pregnancy, risk factors include rubella, and probably influenza, infections in the first or second trimester and antepartum bleeding. At birth, asphyxia and low birth weight, especially with intrauterine growth retardation, are risk factors, as are certain brain insults and infections in childhood.

Early developmental delays

Longitudinal follow-up studies of large birth cohorts have shown that the 1–2% of the sample who go on to develop adult schizophrenia show slight delays in motor, speech and intellectual milestones compared with the rest of the cohort. These differences are subtle, such as walking being delayed by 1–2 months.

Certain problems, such as developmental receptive language disorders, are particularly linked to later schizophrenia. These developmental delays do not occur in bipolar disorder.

Secondary schizophrenias

The so-called secondary schizophrenias fit less easily into the neurodevelopmental formulation. The psychotic symptoms in these cases appear to be caused by a primary, organic disorder: either a known physical disorder or a clinically unsuspected brain lesion.

Table 5.3 lists those medical conditions in which a clear or possible association with schizophrenia-like disorders has been reported. Clinically recommended screening investigations are outlined in Table 5.4.

Street-drug use

Use of cannabis and amphetamine-like drugs has long been known to be an important trigger of relapse, but was thought not to play a truly causal role in the onset of illness. Several cohort studies since 2000

TABLE 5.3

Physical diseases with an increased risk of schizophrenic symptoms

- Epilepsy, temporal lobe
- Infections
    - limbic encephalitis; subacute sclerosing panencephalitis
    - neurosyphilis
    - neurocysticercosis
    - human immunodeficiency virus
- Cerebral trauma
- Cerebrovascular disease (late-onset schizophrenia)
- Demyelinating diseases
    - multiple sclerosis (with temporal plaques)
    - Schilder's disease
    - metachromatic leukodystrophy
- Neurodevelopmental disorders
    - velocardiofacial syndrome

TABLE 5.4

Screening investigations in first-episode schizophrenia

First-line

- Neurological examination
- Complete blood cell count
- Routine blood biochemistry
- Thyroid function
- Liver function
- Electroencephalogram
- Drug screen: urine or hair

Second-line

- Computed tomography/ magnetic resonance imaging
- Autoantibodies
- Serum calcium
- Syphilis serology
- HIV serology
- Chromosome studies
- Serum copper
- Arylsulfatase A
- CSF examination

CSF, cerebrospinal fluid; HIV, human immunodeficiency virus.

have shown that use of cannabis doubles the risk of developing schizophrenia.

The risk is further increased if there are pre-existing minor psychotic symptoms and if cannabis use starts early in adolescence. Subsequent research suggests that this effect of cannabis may be mediated by a particular gene. Those with a specific version of the catechol-O-methyltransferase (*COMT*) gene, carried by about a quarter of the population, appear to be especially prone to psychosis after cannabis use. Delta-9-THC, the active component of cannabis, disrupts learning and recall in schizophrenia.

Psychosocial risk factors

There is emerging evidence for the role of non-biological risk factors in schizophrenia, such as the effects of urban upbringing and of ethnicity, as noted in Chapter 3.

Key points – developmental theories and environmental factors

- Early neurodevelopmental, non-genetic risk factors exist for schizophrenia.
- Birth complications increase the child's risk of schizophrenia in later life fourfold.
- Psychosocial risk factors are being re-established as important risk factors.
- Cannabis use appears to increase the risk of schizophrenia as well as relapse.
- Evidence for specific gene–environment interactions is beginning to emerge.

Key references

Arseneault L, Cannon M, Poulton R et al. Cannabis use in adolescence and risk for adult psychosis: longitudinal prospective study. *BMJ* 2002;325:1212–13.

Bertolino A, Caforio G, Blasi G et al. Interaction of *COMT* (Val(108/158)Met) genotype and olanzapine treatment on prefrontal cortical function in patients with schizophrenia. *Am J Psychiatry* 2004;161:1798–805.

Brown AS, Susser E, Cohen SG, Greenwald S. Schizophrenia following prenatal rubella exposure: gestational timing and diagnostic specificity. *Schizophr Res* 1998;29: 17–18.

Cannon M, Caspi A, Moffitt TE et al. Evidence for early childhood, pandevelopmental impairment specific to schizophreniform disorder: results from a longitudinal birth cohort. *Arch Gen Psychiatry* 2002;59:449–56.

Caspi A, Moffitt TE, Cannon M et al. Moderation of the effect of adolescent-onset cannabis use on adult psychosis by a functional polymorphism in the catechol-O-methyltransferase gene: longitudinal evidence of a gene X environment interaction. *Biol Psychiatry* 2005;57:1117–27.

Henquet C, Murray R, Linszen D, van Os J. The environment and schizophrenia: the role of cannabis use. *Schizophr Bull* 2005;31:608–12.

Hollister JM, Laing P, Mednick SA. Rhesus incompatibility as a risk factor for schizophrenia in male adults. *Arch Gen Psychiatry* 1996;53:19–24.

Howlin P, Mawhood L, Rutter M. Autism and developmental receptive language disorder – a follow-up comparison in early adult life. II: social, behavioural, and psychiatric outcomes. *J Child Psychol Psychiatry* 2000;41:561–78.

Hultman CM, Ohman A, Cnattingius S et al. Prenatal and neonatal risk factors for schizophrenia. *Br J Psychiatry* 1997;170:128–33.

Jones P, Rodgers B, Murray R, Marmot M. Child developmental risk factors for adult schizophrenia in the British 1946 birth cohort. *Lancet* 1994;344:1398–402.

Murray RM, Lewis SW, Reveley AM. Towards an aetiological classification of schizophrenia. *Lancet* 1985; 1:1023–6.

Rantakallio P, Jones P, Moring J, von Wendt L. Association between central nervous system infections during childhood and adult-onset schizophrenia and other psychoses: a 28-year follow-up. *Int J Epidemiol* 1997;26:837–43.

Weinberger DR. Implications of normal brain development for the pathogenesis of schizophrenia. *Arch Gen Psychiatry* 1987;44:660–9.

Our knowledge of the neuroanatomy of schizophrenia is derived from four major sources:

- structural imaging
- neuropsychology and functional imaging
- psychopharmacology
- postmortem neurochemical and structural investigations.

Structural imaging has been the procedure most extensively used to examine the brains of patients with schizophrenia.

Early imaging studies

The first structural imaging studies were performed using pneumoencephalography (PEG), a technique based on the X-ray contrast of air injected into the lumbar subarachnoid space, bone and brain tissue. PEG studies documented a number of abnormalities in patients with schizophrenia, including ventricular system enlargement. However, the invasive nature of the procedure limited its application and eventually led to the abandonment of its use.

The next major development in structural imaging was the introduction of computed tomography (CT), an in vivo, X-ray-based imaging technique for visualizing the brain. The advent of CT scanning enabled investigators to confirm the observation of ventricular enlargement. This finding has been reproduced many times and represents one of the most commonly observed biological findings in schizophrenia. The other major abnormality revealed by CT scanning is a widening of the cortical sulci, which separate the different cerebral gyri.

These observations have greatly influenced our understanding of schizophrenia pathophysiology. They provided strong evidence that a substantial proportion of patients with schizophrenia are characterized by structural abnormalities of the brain. In addition, they helped to reawaken interest in schizophrenia as a brain disease and counteracted the prevailing view at that time of schizophrenia being caused by psychosocial factors.

There are, however, two major limitations to CT scanning. First, CT scans do not permit sufficient resolution of cortical and subcortical gray matter (i.e. nerve cells) and white matter (i.e. fiber tracts connecting different nerve cells). The lack of resolution precludes the morphological assessment of specific cortical and subcortical structures. Second, although ventricular enlargement and cortical sulcal widening suggest that patients with schizophrenia may have relatively less brain tissue than normal controls, they are non-specific measures and cannot tell us where in the brain the tissue loss occurs, or whether the decrease in tissue is due to a developmental failure or to neurodegenerative processes.

There are a number of structures anatomically related to the ventricular system, including basal ganglia nuclei, limbic system structures (i.e. the amygdala and hippocampus), thalamus and cortical white matter. Ventricular enlargement could be due to morphological abnormalities in any one or combination of these structures. Similarly, sulcal widening could be due to changes in cortical gray and/or white matter. Only the direct measurement of these two cortical tissue types would allow the cause of sulcal widening to be determined.

Magnetic resonance imaging

The advent of magnetic resonance imaging (MRI) enabled investigators to overcome the limitations of CT scanning. MRI produces high-quality images, based on the use of magnetic energy and the water content of different tissue types. MRI scans can be segmented into the three different tissue types or compartments:
- gray matter, both cortical and subcortical
- white matter
- cerebrospinal fluid.

These three compartments can each be measured, and for the first time investigators could examine whether patients with schizophrenia were characterized by specific brain morphological abnormalities. MRI scans can also be obtained in a three-dimensional format, from which three-dimensional representations of the brain can be constructed (Figure 6.1). These three-dimensional representations facilitate the morphological assessment of specific cortical gyri.

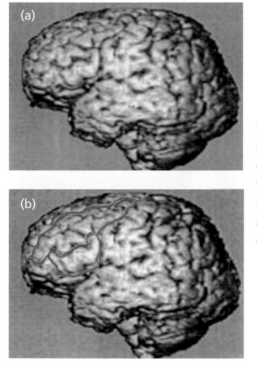

Figure 6.1 (a) A three-dimensional representation of the brain constructed from MRI, with (b) sulcal landmarks for the inferior and middle prefrontal gyri demarcated.

MRI studies were able to confirm the previous findings of enlarged ventricles, with patients exhibiting about a one-third increase in ventricular volume compared with controls (Figure 6.2), and increased sulcal widening (Figure 6.3). MRI studies demonstrated for the first time

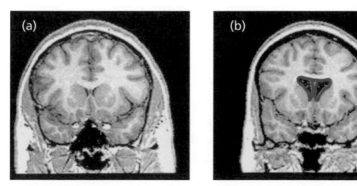

Figure 6.2 MRI scans in the coronal plane of (a) a normal control and (b) a patient with schizophrenia, showing enlarged ventricles.

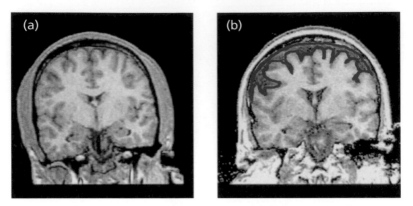

Figure 6.3 MRI scans of (a) a normal control and (b) a patient with schizophrenia, showing increased sulcal widening, which is associated with increased cortical cerebrospinal fluid (shown in the highlighted areas).

the involvement of cortical and subcortical gray matter structures. Specifically, patients with schizophrenia were shown to exhibit decreased volume of the neocortex, by about 5%, with specific gray matter reductions in the prefrontal, superior temporal and inferior parietal heteromodal cortices. These brain regions are the neuroanatomic substrate for the complex cognitive behaviors that are uniquely affected in patients with schizophrenia. In addition to volume reductions in these areas, several studies have found that patients with schizophrenia have a reversal or loss of the normal asymmetry of these structures.

MRI studies have also documented decreased volume of limbic system structures such as the amygdala, hippocampus and parahippocampus (Figure 6.4). These structures are involved in the regulation of emotions and various forms of memory. The magnitude of these changes is relatively small (Table 6.1), but the observations have been shown to be highly reliable, especially for the hippocampus.

Finally, MRI studies have documented a decrease in the volume of specific thalamic nuclei and in the total volume of the thalamus. Thalamic nuclei play a central role in gating the flow of information to the cerebral cortex and in regulating the activation of specific cortical brain areas in response to external or internal stimuli or signals. These MRI results are consistent with postmortem study reports that have

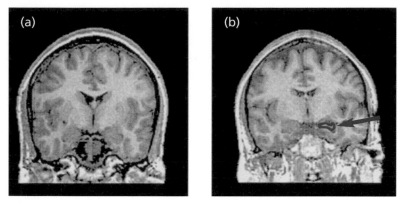

Figure 6.4 MRI scans of (a) a normal control and (b) a patient with schizophrenia with a hippocampus of abnormal shape and volume (see arrow).

documented decreased volume of the medial dorsal and pulvinar thalamic nuclei.

In addition to locating the areas of the brain affected by schizophrenia, MRI studies have also been useful for studying:

- pathophysiological models of schizophrenia
- neuroanatomy of cognitive abnormalities and symptoms
- morphological consequences of exposure to environmental risk factors
- etiologic theories of schizophrenia.

TABLE 6.1

How big are the changes in brain structure in schizophrenia?

Total ventricular volume	Increased	20–30%
Total cranial volume	Decreased	2–4%
Total brain volume	Decreased	2–4%
Heteromodal association cortex (prefrontal superior temporal, inferior parietal cortices)	Decreased	5–10%
Medial temporal lobe (e.g. hippocampus)	Decreased	4–10%
Thalamus	Decreased	5–10%

A series of longitudinal studies involving multiple MRI has evaluated whether schizophrenia is a neurodevelopmental disorder, with fixed morphological abnormalities, or a neurodegenerative disorder, with progressive changes in brain structure. These studies, conducted in childhood-onset, first-episode and chronic patient populations, have consistently demonstrated 2–10% decreases in cortical and subcortical gray matter volumes and 5–10% increases in ventricular volume. The extent to which these results apply to a subgroup or to the total schizophrenia population is unknown. The results, however, are consistent with observations of increased functional disability and progressive neurocognitive impairments in a substantial proportion of patients.

MRI studies have also documented sex differences. Male patients with schizophrenia have been found in some, but not all, studies to have greater reductions in tissue volume, particularly in the temporal lobes. These morphological differences may represent the interaction of the disease process with normal sex differences in brain development and structure, and may provide a structural explanation as to why the course of schizophrenia is frequently more benign in female patients.

Several studies have observed an association between decreased volume of the superior temporal gyrus (STG) gray matter and hallucinations and delusions or positive formal thought disorder. Hallucinations and delusions are more frequently associated with decreased volume of the anterior STG, and positive formal thought disorder with decreased volume of the posterior STG.

MRI has also been used to show that patients with schizophrenia have a loss of the normal asymmetry of the cerebral hemispheres, especially of the planum temporale, a region of the brain involved in audition and language. These observations have led to the development of etiologic hypotheses concerning abnormalities in the normal process of brain lateralization.

Finally, a basic question that has not been adequately addressed is what effect, if any, do antipsychotic agents have on brain structure? And, if they have an effect, does the effect differ between conventional and second-generation antipsychotics? It is hoped that MRI studies, in combination with other imaging techniques, will be able to answer these critical questions.

Diffusion tensor imaging

The observation of multiple morphological abnormalities in cortical and subcortical gray matter raises the question of whether there is a disturbance in the white matter fiber tracts that connect these regions. There have been previous reports of decreased white matter volume, but such changes have not been observed consistently. Moreover, traditional MRI structural scans are not able to differentiate specific fiber tracts.

Diffusion tensor imaging (DTI) is based on the diffusion of water through different brain tissues and allows for the evaluation of white matter integrity. In addition, DTI may be used to identify and measure specific white matter fiber tracts. DTI studies have documented abnormalities in the white matter of patients with schizophrenia, but the localization of the abnormalities has differed across studies. The heterogeneity of findings may reflect the ongoing development of this methodology. Few studies have analyzed specific fiber tracts. The full potential of DTI awaits further refinements in image analytic procedures.

Summary of brain pathology

The reduced cerebral cortical volume and thickness observed with MRI appears to result from a loss of the supportive glial cells, such as astrocytes, leading to an increased packing of neurons (Table 6.2). Glial cells, particularly astrocytes, promote synaptic function. Reduced synaptic and dendritic complexity is seen. These changes might result

TABLE 6.2

Histopathological findings in the cerebral cortex in schizophrenia

- Reduced glial-cell density
- Increased neuronal density
- Aberrant migration of neurons
- Smaller neurons
- Loss of synapses
- Loss of dendritic complexity

from early developmental abnormalities, from abnormal fiber tract connections, from an increase in the synaptic pruning that normally occurs in adolescence or from a later, progressive process.

Key points – neuroanatomy and structural imaging

- Patients with schizophrenia exhibit gray matter reductions in the prefrontal, superior temporal and inferior parietal heteromodal cortices.
- Patients with schizophrenia have decreased volume of subcortical structures, including the amygdala, hippocampus, parahippocampus and thalamus.
- A subgroup of patients may exhibit progressive changes in brain structure over the course of their illness.
- Male patients with schizophrenia have been found to have greater volume reductions in the temporal lobes than female patients.
- Hallucinations, delusions and positive formal thought disorder are associated with decreased volume of the superior temporal gyrus.

Key references

Andreasen NC, Arndt S, Swayze V 2nd et al. Thalamic abnormalities in schizophrenia visualized through magnetic resonance image averaging. *Science* 1994;266:294–8.

Barta PE, Pearlson GD, Brill LB 2nd et al. Planum temporale asymmetry reversal in schizophrenia: replication and relationship to gray matter abnormalities. *Am J Psychiatry* 1997;154:661–7.

Buchanan RW, Breier A, Kirkpatrick B et al. Structural abnormalities in deficit and nondeficit schizophrenia. *Am J Psychiatry* 1993;150:59–65.

Buchanan RW, Francis A, Arango C et al. Morphometric assessment of the heteromodal association cortex in schizophrenia. *Am J Psychiatry* 2004;161:322–31.

Cahn W, Hulshoff Pol HE, Lems EB et al. Brain volume changes in first-episode schizophrenia: a 1-year follow-up study. *Arch Gen Psychiatry* 2002;59:1002–10.

Frederikse M, Lu A, Aylward E et al. Sex differences in inferior parietal lobule volume in schizophrenia. *Am J Psychiatry* 2000;157:422–7.

Gogtay N, Sporn A, Clasen LS et al. Comparison of progressive cortical gray matter loss in childhood-onset schizophrenia with that in childhood-onset atypical psychoses. *Arch Gen Psychiatry* 2004;61:17–22.

Kanaan RA, Kim JS, Kaufmann WE et al. Diffusion tensor imaging in schizophrenia. *Biol Psychiatry* 2005;58:921–9.

Lieberman JA, Tollefson GD, Charles C et al. Antipsychotic drug effects on brain morphology in first-episode psychosis. *Arch Gen Psychiatry* 2005;62:361–70.

Lim KO, Hedehus M, Moseley M et al. Compromised white matter tract integrity in schizophrenia inferred from diffusion tensor imaging. *Arch Gen Psychiatry* 1999;56:367–74.

Mathalon DH, Sullivan EV, Lim KO, Pfefferbaum A. Progressive brain volume changes and the clinical course of schizophrenia in men: a longitudinal magnetic resonance imaging study. *Arch Gen Psychiatry* 2001;58:148–57.

Pearlson GD, Petty RG, Ross CA, Tien AY. Schizophrenia: a disease of heteromodal association cortex? *Neuropsychopharmacology* 1996; 14:1–17.

Shenton ME, Dickey CC, Frumin M, McCarley RW. A review of MRI findings in schizophrenia. *Schizophr Res* 2001;49:1–52.

Wright IC, Rabe-Hesketh S, Woodruff PW et al. Meta-analysis of regional brain volumes in schizophrenia. *Am J Psychiatry* 2000;157:16–25.

The original name for schizophrenia, dementia praecox, reflects the appreciation of even the earliest investigators of the primary role of neurocognitive impairments in schizophrenia. However, the precise nature and extent of these impairments remain unknown. Are there specific, fundamental impairments that all patients share and that are responsible for the broad range of neurocognitive abnormalities observed in schizophrenia, or do the multiple abnormalities reflect the widespread pathophysiological involvement of the brain? When do neurocognitive impairments first become manifest, and under what circumstances do they progress? What is the relationship of neurocognitive impairments to other aspects of schizophrenia?

Neurocognitive impairments

What is their nature? Patients with schizophrenia present with a broad range of neurocognitive impairments. Many of these impairments may be detected through the use of traditional neuropsychological assessments and include abnormalities in processing speed, reasoning and problem solving, verbal and visual learning and memory, working memory and social cognition (Table 7.1). These domains of impairment may reflect abnormalities in more basic cognitive functions, which can be detected through the use of sophisticated neurocognitive paradigms. For example, recent studies of visual information processing have demonstrated subtle impairments in early sensory information processing, which may contribute to impaired performance on more complex neuropsychological tasks.

In addition to impairments on neuropsychological measures of cognitive function, patients with schizophrenia also exhibit impairments in cognitive functions assessed through the use of sophisticated computerized assessment procedures. These techniques are able to detect basic information processing (referred to above), eye-tracking and sensory gating abnormalities. There are two major types of eye-tracking

TABLE 7.1

Core cognitive impairments in schizophrenia

Cognitive domain	Tests of domain
Attention/information processing	Continuous Performance Test
Processing speed	WAIS-III Digit Span, Trails A, Category Fluency
Reasoning and problem solving	WAIS-III Block Design, Wisconsin Card Sort, Tower of London
Verbal learning and memory	WAIS-III Logical Memory, California Verbal Learning Test, Hopkins Verbal Learning Test
Visual learning and memory	WMS-III Visual Reproduction, Brief Visuospatial Test
Working memory	WAIS-III Letter–Number Sequencing, N-Back Test
Social cognition	Penn Emotional Recognition Test, Penn Emotional Acuity Test

WAIS, Wechsler Adult Intelligence Scale; WMS, Wechsler Memory Scale.

abnormality: one involves the smooth-pursuit eye movement system and is reflected in an inability to track objects as they move through space, whereas the other involves the saccadic eye movement system, which is used to correct the gaze of subjects when they have moved off target. Patients with schizophrenia are less able to inhibit inappropriate saccadic eye movement intrusions into their smooth-pursuit eye movements, and are less able to produce saccadic eye movements in the direction opposite to a visual stimulus.

Two forms of sensory gating abnormality have been extensively examined in patients with schizophrenia: P50 and prepulse inhibition (PPI). Normal individuals are able to gradually ignore repetitive stimuli, whereas patients with schizophrenia experience each stimulus as a novel stimulus and are unable to suppress their response to the repetitive sensory stimuli. This abnormality is thought to be related to the heightened distractibility that afflicts patients with schizophrenia.

The P50 evoked-potential paradigm is used to detect the presence of this abnormality. PPI refers to the diminishment of a startle response to a stimulus, when a less intense form of the stimulus (the prepulse stimulus) is presented prior to the full stimulus. Patients with schizophrenia fail to respond to the prepulse stimulus with decreased startle response. P50 and PPI abnormalities may be reversed by some antipsychotic medications, nicotine and other pharmacological agents.

Studies of families and twins suggest that several of these neurocognitive impairments may not only be characteristic features of schizophrenia, but may also be present in non-affected family members. In particular, abnormalities of attention, verbal memory, eye-tracking and P50 have been shown to occur at a higher-than-expected rate in family members than in the general population. These observations have led to the supposition that these impairments may represent alternative phenotypic markers of the illness (see Chapter 4).

When do they occur? The results of high-risk and large-scale birth cohort studies and studies of military inductees who have gone on to develop schizophrenia provide compelling evidence that patients with schizophrenia exhibit subtle neurocognitive impairments prior to the onset of more florid psychotic symptoms. These impairments may be present in early childhood and are already present in patients who are experiencing their first episode of schizophrenia (Table 7.2).

TABLE 7.2

Neurocognitive deficits present in the first episode

- Attention/vigilance
- Executive function
- Fine motor function
- Processing speed
- Spatial working memory
- Verbal learning and memory

Studies of IQ test scores obtained routinely during childhood show that those children who will later develop schizophrenia have slightly, but significantly, lower mean scores than do either age- and social-class-matched normal children or siblings. The most convincing studies have been those of large, unselected birth cohorts that were followed and tested at regular intervals. At the time of onset of positive psychotic symptoms, there is usually a further decline in cognitive function. Patients will typically exhibit a five- to ten-point decline in their IQ score.

What is the pathophysiology? Neurocognitive impairments may reflect the involvement of specific brain regions or neural circuits, or they may reflect a more global involvement of the brain. There is evidence for both hypotheses.

The pattern of predominant impairments suggests the relatively selective involvement of frontotemporal areas. The results of functional imaging studies are also consistent with the selective involvement of frontotemporal areas, although this may be due in part to the nature of the cognitive tasks studied. These studies also implicate the hippocampus in the pathophysiology of these impairments.

On the other hand, the pattern of predominant impairments may be more apparent than real. Several studies suggest that the cognitive impairments in patients are highly correlated with each other and that patient/normal control differences are largely due to differences in general intelligence. The question of whether there are a few basic cognitive abnormalities that underlie the broad range of observed cognitive manifestations or whether multiple cognitive processes are independently affected in schizophrenia, is a basic unresolved issue.

What is the relationship with other aspects of schizophrenia? The relationship between cognitive impairments and individual symptom clusters and other domains of schizophrenia psychopathology has been the focus of extensive investigation. Patients with negative symptoms and symptoms of behavioral disorganization are more likely to exhibit clinically significant neurocognitive impairments than are patients without these symptoms.

Several studies have suggested that negative symptoms are selectively associated with impaired performance on neuropsychological measures sensitive to lesions of the frontal or parietal lobes. Patients with negative symptoms have also been shown to be the most impaired on tasks requiring self-generated, rather than stimulus-driven, activity. In contrast, disorganized patients are characterized by impaired performance on measures of distractibility, and they are also more likely to show an inability to inhibit inappropriate behavioral responses.

Patients with schizophrenia are characterized by poor social and occupational functioning. There has been a growing appreciation of the central role that neurocognitive impairments play in the development of these functional disabilities. Impairments of verbal memory, language, vigilance and executive function have been shown to be determinants of poor social and community function. Impairments of memory and executive and processing speed have been related to poor occupational outcome.

The relationship of neurocognitive impairments to the broad range of symptom and functional outcomes suggests that the development of effective treatments for these impairments would have far-reaching beneficial effects on patients with schizophrenia.

Functional imaging

Whatever else underlies the symptoms and deficits of schizophrenia, there is plainly a disturbance of brain function. Schizophrenia research has, therefore, been quick to use imaging techniques that demonstrate disturbances in brain function. However, it was not until the late 1970s that neuroscientists came to believe that, just as in other tissues (e.g. muscle), the blood flow and metabolism of brain tissue increased when a region was specifically active.

The invention of imaging techniques that are able to show regional cerebral blood flow or metabolism confirmed that the blood flow to regions of primary motor or sensory cortex increases by 5–10% a few seconds after movement or perception begins. Similar changes of lesser magnitude also occur in brain regions executing a complex cognitive task, such as solving a puzzle. These changes can be used to clarify which areas of the brain are being used to do specific tasks.

PET, SPECT, BOLD and MRS. The main functional imaging techniques are outlined in Table 7.3.

Positron emission tomography (PET) and single-photon emission computed tomography (SPECT) were the first true functional brain-scanning techniques. They both rely on intravenous injection or inhalation of radioactive tracers, which are taken up into the brain in proportion to local blood flow and produce a map of glucose metabolism or regional cerebral blood flow (rCBF). PET uses

TABLE 7.3

Comparison of functional brain imaging techniques

	SPECT	PET	fMR	MRS
Availability	+++	+	+++	++
Safety	+	++	+++	+++
Spatial resolution	6 mm	3 mm	3 mm	5 mm
Time resolution	Hours	Minutes	Seconds	Minutes
Sensitivity	+	+++	++	++
Parameters measured	Regional cerebral blood flow Receptor density and binding	Regional cerebral blood flow Receptor density Glucose metabolism	Regional cerebral blood flow	Selected biochemistry (e.g. phosphate)
Drawbacks	High radiation levels	Expensive	Sensitive to movement artifact	Strong magnetic fields are best

fMR, functional magnetic resonance; MRS, magnetic resonance spectroscopy; PET, positron-emission tomography; SPECT, single-photon emission computed tomography.
+, little advantage for this technique; ++, moderate advantage for this technique; +++, strong advantage for this technique.

radioactive isotopes with short half-lives, which limits the amount of radiation received and enables repeated measurements in one session. PET isotopes decay to release two gamma rays, or photons, whereas SPECT isotopes emit just one photon at a time. In each case, the photons are recorded by detectors arrayed around the head. PET is superior to SPECT because smaller changes can be detected and more accurately pinpointed.

Functional magnetic resonance imaging (fMRI). The safest and most widely used technique is functional magnetic resonance (fMR) blood-oxygen-level-dependent (BOLD) imaging. This produces a map of rCBF and brain activity from the natural change in paramagnetic properties of hemoglobin as it deoxygenates. Initial problems of low resolution and movement artifacts with fMR have been overcome, and this is now the most widely applied functional imaging approach.

Magnetic resonance spectroscopy (MRS) allows the assessment of brain biochemistry. [31]Phosphorus MRS shows a series of peaks, which correspond to energy reactions in the cell, involving adenosine triphosphate, as well as turnover of membranes in synapses and vesicles (Figure 7.1).

In untreated schizophrenia, MRS of the prefrontal cortex has repeatedly shown a decrease in phosphomonoesters and an increase in

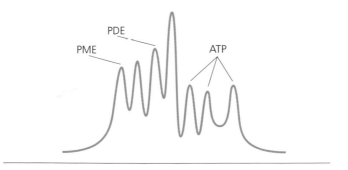

PDE

PME

ATP

Chemical shift

Figure 7.1 [31]Phosphorus magnetic resonance spectroscopy for assessment of brain biochemistry. ATP, adenosine triphosphate; PDE, phosphodiesters; PME, phosphomonoesters.

phosphodiesters. This suggests a decreased synthesis and/or increased breakdown of cell membrane phospholipids, which might reflect disturbed pruning of synapses. Proton MRS visualizes a separate set of biochemical processes and suggests reduced frontal glutamate activity in early schizophrenia.

One current hypothesis suggests that this reduced glutamate activity turns into increased activity at the onset of the illness, with excitatory damage leading to synaptic loss and longer-term progression of the illness.

Experimental design

Imaging brain function is more difficult than imaging brain structure. Ensuring that patients and controls are engaged in similar standardized cognitive activity is usually important, to reduce chance variations and allow real differences to be seen. Unless they are properly controlled for, drug effects can mask all other effects.

A common method of investigating the abnormal brain function underpinning a cognitive deficit is to first scan a normal subject before and during the execution of a relevant task. By subtracting the brain activity map as it was before the task from the map during the task, the specific areas of the brain involved in the task will be highlighted. The same brain activity maps are then produced for schizophrenia patients before and during the same task, which can then be compared with the pattern in normal subjects. A general finding is that patients with schizophrenia tend to use aberrant networks of cortical activity, even during simple cognitive, perceptual or motor tasks and even when performance is apparently normal.

Image analysis is challenging. There are two general approaches. In the top-down 'region of interest' approach, functional images have to be mapped precisely onto structural scans ('coregistration'). More widely used is the bottom-up 'voxel-based morphometry', where images from groups of subjects, or the same subjects during and after a cognitive challenge, are transformed into identical brain shapes with differences between groups then expressed as maps of significant p-value scores (e.g. those of $p < 0.01$). This is called statistical parametric mapping.

Mapping symptoms

Functional imaging has been informative at the level of understanding individual symptoms, symptom clusters and specific cognitive deficits in schizophrenia (Figure 7.2). The three overlapping syndromes outlined in Chapter 2 correlate with particular cognitive deficits and with distinct patterns of brain function (Tables 7.4 and 7.5).

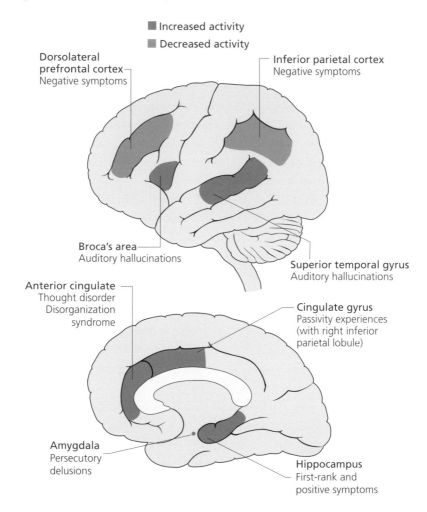

Figure 7.2 The localization of psychotic symptoms and deficits in the brain, as shown by functional imaging studies: (a) lateral view of left hemisphere; (b) medial view of left hemisphere.

TABLE 7.4

Functional imaging: how symptoms and brain activity correlate

Symptom	Brain regions involved	Activity change (vs normal)
Negative symptoms/ psychomotor poverty	Left dorsolateral prefrontal cortex	Decrease
	Inferior parietal cortex	Decrease
Auditory hallucinations	Broca's area	Increase
	Superior temporal gyrus (left)	Fails to decrease
Total positive symptoms	Hippocampal region	Increase
Formal thought disorder	Anterior cingulate	Increase
	Superior temporal gyrus (left)	Decrease
Persecutory delusions	Amygdala	Increase
Passivity experiences	Cingulate gyrus	Increase
	Right parietal lobule	Increase

TABLE 7.5

Functional imaging of cognitive deficits in schizophrenia

Cognitive deficit in	Failure of normal activation in
Working memory	Left inferior prefrontal cortex
	Medial temporal cortex
Verbal fluency	Left dorsolateral prefrontal cortex
	Failure to deactivate superior temporal cortex
Error monitoring	Anterior cingulate gyrus
Facial emotion recognition	Amygdala
Olfaction	Insula
	Parahippocampal gyrus
Inhibition of reflex eye saccades	Striatum

> **Key points – neuropsychology and functional imaging**
>
> - Patients with schizophrenia exhibit subtle neurocognitive impairments prior to the onset of florid psychotic symptoms.
> - Studies of families and twins suggest that several neurocognitive impairments may be present in non-affected family members.
> - Neurocognitive impairments are a major determinant of poor social and occupational functioning.
> - Positive psychotic symptoms correlate with hippocampal activation.
> - Negative symptoms correlate with decreased activity in the dorsolateral prefrontal cortex.
> - The disorganization syndrome correlates with increased activity in the anterior cingulate gyrus.

Negative symptoms, or the psychomotor poverty syndrome, correlate with decreased activity in the dorsolateral prefrontal cortex, particularly on the left. Interestingly, this pattern also appears in severe depressive illness with psychomotor retardation, thus indicating a final common cortical deficit underlying psychomotor poverty in schizophrenia and psychomotor retardation in depression. Positive psychotic symptoms correlate with hippocampal activation and with a distributed network of frontal, temporal and subcortical sites. The disorganization syndrome correlates with increased activity in the dorsal anterior cingulate gyrus, a region involved in selective attention.

Among positive symptoms, auditory hallucinations, rather than delusions, have been most extensively studied. This is partly because the normal cerebral mechanisms of auditory perception are well understood, but the normal mechanisms underlying the formation of beliefs are not. During auditory hallucinations, increased blood flow is seen in Broca's area in the left hemisphere. This is similar to the activity produced during normal speech and during normal 'inner' speech, when one is rehearsing something silently to oneself. In a healthy brain, a connected area of cortex in the superior temporal gyrus is deactivated during inner speech. Functional imaging shows that this does not occur in hallucinating patients, suggesting that hallucinations may actually be misinterpreted inner speech.

In some cases, the link between a specific symptom and a functional abnormality emerges only under particular conditions. Compared with controls, patients with persecutory delusions show increased activation in the amygdala in situations of possible threat. Patients with auditory hallucinations show right-sided temporoparietal and parahippocampal deficits during inner speech tasks, which again suggest an internal monitoring problem.

Key references

Achim AM, Lepage M. Episodic memory-related activation in schizophrenia: meta-analysis. *Br J Psychiatry* 2005;187:500–9.

Bilder RM, Goldman RS, Robinson D et al. Neuropsychology of first-episode schizophrenia: initial characterization and clinical correlates. *Am J Psychiatry* 2000;157:549–59.

Buchanan RW, Strauss ME, Kirkpatrick B et al. Neuropsychological impairments in deficit vs nondeficit forms of schizophrenia. *Arch Gen Psychiatry* 1994;51: 804–11.

Cairo TA, Woodward TS, Ngan ET. Decreased encoding efficiency in schizophrenia. *Biol Psychiatry* 2006;59:740–6.

Crespo-Facorro B, Paradiso S, Andreasen NC et al. Neural mechanisms of anhedonia in schizophrenia: a PET study of response to unpleasant and pleasant odors. *JAMA* 2001;286:427–35.

Dickinson D, Iannone VN, Wilk CM, Gold JM. General and specific cognitive deficits in schizophrenia. *Biol Psychiatry* 2004;55:826–33.

Freedman R, Adler LE, Myles-Worsley M et al. Inhibitory gating of an evoked response to repeated auditory stimuli in schizophrenic and normal subjects. Human recordings, computer simulation, and an animal model. *Arch Gen Psychiatry* 1996;53: 1114–21.

Frith CD, Friston KJ, Herold S et al. Regional brain activity in chronic schizophrenic patients during the performance of a verbal fluency task. *Br J Psychiatry* 1995;167:343–9.

Geyer MA, Krebs-Thomson K, Braff DL, Swerdlow NR. Pharmacological studies of prepulse inhibition models of sensorimotor gating deficits in schizophrenia: a decade in review. *Psychopharmacology (Berl)* 2001; 156:117–54.

Green MF, Kern RS, Heaton RK. Longitudinal studies of cognition and functional outcome in schizophrenia: implications for MATRICS. *Schizophr Res* 2004;72:41–51.

Kircher TT, Liddle PF, Brammer MJ et al. Neural correlates of formal thought disorder in schizophrenia: preliminary findings from a functional magnetic resonance imaging study. *Arch Gen Psychiatry* 2001;58:769–74

Liddle PF, Friston KJ, Frith CD et al. Patterns of cerebral blood flow in schizophrenia. *Br J Psychiatry* 1992;160:179–86.

McGuire PK, Silbersweig DA, Wright I et al. Abnormal monitoring of inner speech: a physiological basis for auditory hallucinations. *Lancet* 1995;346:596–600.

Norman RM, Malla AK, Morrison-Stewart SL et al. Neuropsychological correlates of syndromes in schizophrenia. *Br J Psychiatry* 1997;170:134–9.

Nuechterlein KH, Barch DM, Gold JM et al. Identification of separable cognitive factors in schizophrenia. *Schizophr Res* 2004;72:29–39.

Raemaekers M, Ramsey NF, Vink M et al. Brain activation during antisaccades in unaffected relatives of schizophrenic patients. *Biol Psychiatry* 2006;59:530–5.

Saykin AJ, Shtasel DL, Gur RE et al. Neuropsychological deficits in neuroleptic naive patients with first-episode schizophrenia. *Arch Gen Psychiatry* 1994;51:124–31.

Spence SA, Brooks DJ, Hirsch SR et al. A PET study of voluntary movements in schizophrenic patients experiencing passivity phenomena (delusions of alien control). *Brain* 1997;120:1997–2011.

Tek C, Gold J, Blaxton T et al. Visual perceptual and working memory impairments in schizophrenia. *Arch Gen Psychiatry* 2002;59:146–53.

Thaker GK, Ross DE, Cassady SL et al. Saccadic eye movement abnormalities in relatives of patients with schizophrenia. *Schizophr Res* 2000;45:235–44.

Neurochemical abnormalities are the link between underlying causal factors, either genetic or environmental, and the overt expression of signs and symptoms of the illness. Over the last four decades, multiple neurotransmitter systems have been hypothesized to be involved in the neurochemistry of schizophrenia. These hypotheses have fallen in and out of vogue as our knowledge of the brain and our methods for investigating brain neurobiology have become more sophisticated. The major neurochemical pathophysiological hypotheses continue to involve the traditional neurotransmitters, although this situation will likely change over the next decade as findings emerge from the application of novel molecular biological techniques to the study of schizophrenia.

The dopamine hypothesis

Dopamine cell bodies exist in two areas: the hypothalamus and the midbrain. In the hypothalamus, dopamine controls pituitary prolactin release (tuberohypophyseal pathway). The midbrain is the source of three pathways: one from the substantia nigra to the dorsal striatum in the basal ganglia (nigrostriatal pathway), and two others projecting from the ventral tegmental area to the ventral striatum (mesolimbic pathway) and to the frontal cortex (mesocortical pathway) (Figure 8.1).

In the early 1960s, Arvid Carlsson posited the dopamine hypothesis of schizophrenia, in which he stated that schizophrenia was due to an excess of dopaminergic activity: an excess of dopamine release and/or hypersensitivity of dopamine receptors. The hypothesis was supported by several observations. First was the recognition of a schizophrenia-like psychosis in people who misused amphetamine, a drug known to increase the release of dopamine. Second was the emergence of adverse effects of the recently discovered antipsychotic chlorpromazine, which mimicked Parkinson's disease, itself thought to be due to faulty dopamine transmission. Third was the observation that all drugs that were effective antipsychotic agents were dopamine receptor antagonists. In the following 15 years, several experiments have provided

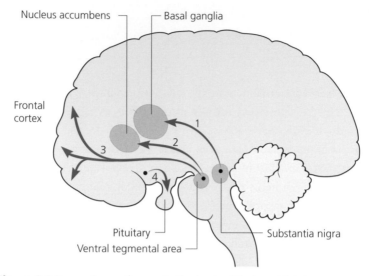

Figure 8.1 Dopamine pathways in the brain: (1) nigrostriatal; (2) mesolimbic; (3) mesocortical; (4) tuberohypophyseal.

compelling, but circumstantial, evidence in further support of the importance of the dopamine D_2 receptor in schizophrenia. However, there were known shortcomings in the dopamine hypothesis and direct evidence was lacking. In addition, the prediction that untreated patients should have increased numbers of dopamine receptors received no firm support from postmortem assays nor, more critically, from studies using positron emission tomography, which imaged the binding of radiolabeled antipsychotic drugs to receptors.

Four developments helped to revive the dopamine hypothesis. First, the hypothesis was reformulated to predict the existence of both hyperdopaminergic and hypodopaminergic activity in schizophrenic patients. Positive symptoms are due to increased activity of the mesolimbic dopamine pathway, whereas negative symptoms are due to decreased activity of the mesocortical dopamine pathway (see Figure 8.1).

Second, in the late 1980s, new biomolecular techniques found five dopamine receptor subtypes. They differ functionally and in their pattern of target neuron/brain region distribution (Table 8.1). D_1 receptors are the most common and are always postsynaptic. D_5 is related. The

TABLE 8.1

Target neuron location of dopamine receptor subtypes

Location	Receptor subtype
Basal ganglia	D_1, D_2
Nucleus accumbens	D_2, D_3
Frontal cortex, hippocampus	D_1, D_4, D_5

D_2 family includes D_2, D_3 and D_4. D_2 receptors are located both presynaptically on dopamine terminals, where they act as autoreceptors regulating dopamine release, and postsynaptically. The development of more specific receptor ligands may lead to new information on the location and role of the different dopamine receptors.

Third, more informative functional imaging approaches have been developed for assessing in vivo dopamine activity. One approach is based on the infusion of indirect dopamine agonists. The extent to which radioligand occupancy of postsynaptic dopamine receptors is reduced by competition with the increased endogenous dopamine is then determined. The comparison of pre- and postinfusion radioligand occupancy provides an index of dopamine release and reuptake rates. Studies using this approach have documented increased dopamine release in patients with schizophrenia compared with normal controls, and suggest that the extent of dopamine release is associated with the severity of positive psychotic symptoms. The other approach has examined the relationship of dopamine D_2 receptor occupancy of antipsychotic medications and the occurrence of symptom remission and adverse effects. These studies have shown a strong association among dopamine D_2 receptor occupancy, antipsychotic dose, symptom remission and adverse effects.

Finally, multiple studies have demonstrated that dopamine plays a central role in reward mechanisms, especially the mesolimbic projection to the nucleus accumbens. Patients with schizophrenia exhibit several impairments that are consistent with altered reward system function, including anhedonia, decreased motivation and failure to use feedback to enhance goal-directed behavior.

Although the dopamine hypothesis remains the most salient hypothesis, there is still the issue that a substantial proportion of patients with schizophrenia do not adequately respond to dopamine antagonists, which suggests that other neurotransmitters are involved in the pathophysiology of schizophrenia.

Does serotonin play a role?

Serotonergic neurons project from the Raphé nucleus in the brainstem to basal ganglia, limbic, thalamic and cortical regions throughout the brain (Figure 8.2). As with dopamine, several families of serotonin (5-HT) receptors have now been identified (Table 8.2). 5-HT was proposed as an important transmitter in schizophrenia before the dopamine hypothesis, mainly because of the psychotomimetic properties of lysergic acid diethylamide, which releases 5-HT. However, no direct supporting evidence has been found; only recently, in the light of the potent 5-HT_{2a} receptor antagonism of clozapine and the other second-generation antipsychotics, have 5-HT mechanisms been seriously considered.

The ratio of 5-HT_{2a} to D_2 blockade has been proposed as the critical distinction between conventional and second-generation antipsychotic

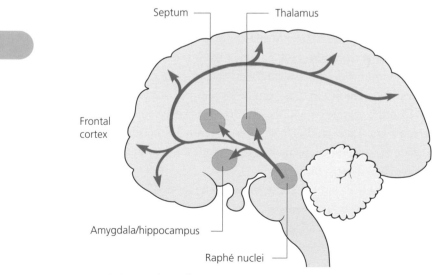

Figure 8.2 Serotonin pathways in the brain.

TABLE 8.2

Human brain serotonin (5-HT) receptors and their actions

Receptor	Action
5-HT$_1$	5-HT$_{1a}$ receptors: involved in anxiolytic/antidepressant actions; may be involved in cognition
	5-HT$_{1b}$ receptors: involved in aggression
	5-HT$_{1d}$ and 5-HT$_{1e}$ receptors: functional role unclear
	5-HT$_{1f}$ receptors: involved in migraine
5-HT$_2$	5-HT$_{2a}$ receptors: modulate ascending dopamine pathways
	5-HT$_{2c}$ receptors: involved in hunger
5-HT$_3$	Found in limbic and frontal cortex May be involved in aggression
5-HT$_4$	May be involved in cognition and anxiety
5-HT$_5$	Functional role unclear
5-HT$_6$	May be involved in cognition and depression
5HT$_7$	May be involved in circadian rhythm and epilepsy

drugs (see Chapter 9 for a review of these drugs). The affinity of clozapine for the 5-HT$_{2a}$ receptor exceeds its affinity for D$_2$ receptors 20-fold, although some conventional antipsychotics, such as chlorpromazine, also have greater affinity for the 5-HT$_{2a}$ receptor than for the D$_2$ receptor. One possible explanation of the therapeutic role of 5-HT$_{2a}$ blockade is that it stimulates dopamine activity in the mesocortical pathways without causing the mesolimbic stimulation that underlies positive symptoms.

Postmortem studies have suggested fewer 5-HT$_{2a}$ receptors in the frontal and temporal cortex, and reduced 5-HT$_{2a}$ gene expression in the frontal cortex, in patients with schizophrenia compared with normal controls. However, treatment studies with selective 5-HT$_{2a}$ antagonists have not been encouraging, and functional imaging studies with 5-HT ligands have not been able to consistently replicate the observation of decreased 5-HT$_{2a}$ receptors in the prefrontal cortex.

The roles of other serotonergic receptors have not been extensively studied, although the 5-HT_{1a}, 5-HT_4 and 5-HT_6 receptors may be promising targets for cognitive-enhancing drugs.

Possible role of glutamate?

Glutamate is the major excitatory neurotransmitter in the central nervous system and plays a central role in cortical–subcortical and thalamic–cortical excitatory projections. Glutamate acts at both ionotropic and metabotropic receptors (Table 8.3). Ionotropic receptors mediate fast excitatory neurotransmission, whereas metabotropic receptors activate second messenger systems through the G-protein system and regulate the release of glutamate and other neuro-transmitters.

TABLE 8.3

Glutamatergic receptors

Ionotropic receptors		Function
NMDA		Neurodevelopment
		Neural plasticity
		Learning and memory
AMPA		Learning and memory
Kainate		Learning and memory

Metabotropic receptors		Localization
Group I	mGlu1	Postsynaptic
	mGlu5	Postsynaptic
Group II	mGlu2	Pre- and postsynaptic
	mGlu3	Pre- and postsynaptic
Group III	mGlu4	Pre- and postsynaptic
	mGlu6	Postsynaptic
	mGlu7	Pre- and postsynaptic
	mGlu8	Pre- and postsynaptic

AMPA, α-amino-3-hydroxy-5-methyl-4-isoxazole propionic acid;
NMDA, N-methyl-D-aspartate.

The N-methyl-D-aspartate (NMDA) and other ionotropic receptors have been most extensively studied in schizophrenia. Abnormalities in NMDA receptor function have been hypothesized to disrupt glutamatergic system function in patients with schizophrenia. There is indirect evidence to support this hypothesis. Phencyclidine (PCP) causes a psychosis that has been described as including positive and negative symptoms and cognitive impairments. PCP exerts its effect through blocking the ion channel gated by the NMDA receptor, which would initially produce a hypoglutamatergic state. However, the PCP-induced decrease in NMDA receptor function may also result in a compensatory glutamatergic hyperactivity in cortical brain regions. In addition, long-term PCP administration results in depletion of prefrontal dopamine. One or more of these diverse effects may underlie the broad range of effects observed with NMDA receptor blockade.

There is accumulating evidence to support a glutamate hypothesis. Postmortem studies have documented abnormal NMDA, α-amino-3-hydroxy-5-methyl-4-isoxazole propionic acid (AMPA) and kainate receptor binding in the prefrontal and temporal cortex, and abnormal NMDA and AMPA messenger RNA receptor expression in the hippocampus. Perhaps the most compelling evidence comes from clinical trials that have examined the efficacy of agents that modify the activity of the NMDA receptor. These studies have shown that glycine, D-serine and D-cycloserine, which bind to the glycine site of the NMDA receptor, and sarcosine, which inhibits glycine reuptake, may be effective treatments for negative symptoms (glycine and D-cycloserine) and positive and negative symptoms (D-serine and sarcosine).

What about acetylcholine?

Acetylcholine acts at muscarinic and nicotinic cholinergic receptors. These receptors are broadly distributed throughout the brain, including the neocortex, hippocampus and basal ganglia. Acetylcholine modulates the release of a number of different neurotransmitters, including dopamine and glutamate. The M_1 muscarinic receptor and the $\alpha_4\beta_2$ and α_7 nicotinic receptors may be particularly important in the regulation of cognitive functions. Cholinergic mechanisms have been implicated in the regulation of attention, memory, processing speed and sensory gating processes – processes which are impaired in patients with schizophrenia. Furthermore, acute nicotine administration has been shown to improve attention, eye-tracking and sensory gating, as measured by P50 or prepulse inhibition, in patients with schizophrenia. Future studies are required to delineate the role of acetylcholine in schizophrenia.

The GABA system?

γ-Aminobutyric acid (GABA) receptors are extensively located on cerebral cortical interneurons and regulate cortical glutamatergic efferents. GABA receptors are also important in processing thalamic inputs to the cerebral cortex. GABA interneurons may be decreased in patients with schizophrenia, with a possible selective decrease in $GABA_A$ receptors. Decreased GABAergic function may contribute to altered cortical function and the broad array of observed cognitive impairments.

Other neurotransmitters

Norepinephrine and neuropeptides are additional neurotransmitters that have been hypothesized to be involved in the pathophysiology of schizophrenia. The multitude of neurochemical hypotheses points to both the possibility of multiple neurotransmitter systems being affected and the lack of definitive evidence for any one system.

Key points – neurochemistry

- The dopamine hypothesis remains the major neurochemical hypothesis of schizophrenia.
- Positive symptoms are hypothesized to be due to increased activity of the mesolimbic dopamine pathway.
- Negative symptoms are hypothesized to be due to decreased activity of the mesocortical dopamine pathway.
- Altered glutamate activity may be involved in the pathophysiology of negative and positive symptoms and cognitive impairments.
- Disturbances in the cholinergic and GABAergic systems have been hypothesized to underlie cognitive impairments in schizophrenia.

Key references

Carlsson A, Waters N, Carlsson ML. Neurotransmitter interactions in schizophrenia – therapeutic implications. *Biol Psychiatry* 1999;46:1388–95.

Farber NB, Newcomer JW, Olney JW. Glycine agonists: what can they teach us about schizophrenia? *Arch Gen Psychiatry* 1999;56:13–17.

Kapur S, Zipursky R, Jones C et al. Relationship between dopamine D(2) occupancy, clinical response, and side effects: a double-blind PET study of first-episode schizophrenia. *Am J Psychiatry* 2000;157:514–20.

Lewis DA, Volk DW, Hashimoto T. Selective alterations in prefrontal cortical GABA neurotransmission in schizophrenia: a novel target for the treatment of working memory dysfunction. *Psychopharmacology (Berl)* 2004;174:143–50.

Moghaddam B. Targeting metabotropic glutamate receptors for treatment of the cognitive symptoms of schizophrenia. *Psychopharmacology (Berl)* 2004;174:39–44.

Roth BL, Hanizavareh SM, Blum AE. Serotonin receptors represent highly favorable molecular targets for cognitive enhancement in schizophrenia and other disorders. *Psychopharmacology (Berl)* 2004;174:17–24.

Schultz W. Predictive reward signal of dopamine neurons. *J Neurophysiol* 1998;80:1 27.

The modern era of pharmacological treatment of schizophrenia began in the early 1950s with the discovery that chlorpromazine (thorazine) had antipsychotic properties. The introduction and eventual widespread use of chlorpromazine and other antipsychotics has facilitated a major paradigm shift in the treatment of the patient with schizophrenia, from a hospital-based to a community-based system of care.

There are two major classes of antipsychotic medications: conventional, traditional or typical antipsychotics or neuroleptics; and second-generation, novel or atypical antipsychotics. Antipsychotic medications constitute the primary class of drugs used to treat schizophrenia.

Conventional antipsychotics

The majority of conventional antipsychotics have a similar mechanism of action, and they are all potent dopamine D_2 receptor antagonists. This property is hypothesized to be the basis of their antipsychotic action. There are five major classes of these drugs (Table 9.1).

There are both oral and injectable, long-acting depot forms of antipsychotics. Their primary indication is for positive symptoms, such as hallucinations, delusions and positive formal thought disorder. They have limited efficacy for negative symptoms or cognitive impairments in patients with schizophrenia.

In the treatment of acute psychotic episodes, these drugs will usually begin to improve symptoms within the first week. Improvement will continue to accrue over the following few months of treatment, with most improvement occurring during the first 6 weeks of treatment. The usual dosage of a conventional antipsychotic for the treatment of an acute episode should be in the range of 300–1000 chlorpromazine equivalents (CPZE)/day, where 100 CPZE is the dose equivalent to 100 mg of chlorpromazine (Table 9.1).

Conventional antipsychotics are also indicated for the maintenance phase of treatment. Maintenance treatment is designed to suppress psychotic symptomatology and/or prevent the reoccurrence of a

TABLE 9.1

Conventional antipsychotics

Class	Generic name	Chlorpromazine equivalents of commonly used drugs
Phenothiazines	Chlorpromazine	100 mg
	Mesoridazine*	50 mg
	Thioridazine*	100 mg
	Fluphenazine	2 mg
	Perphenazine	10 mg
	Trifluoperazine	5 mg
Thioxanthenes	Thiothixene*	5 mg
Butyrophenones	Haloperidol	2 mg
Dibenzoxazepines	Loxapine*	10 mg
Dihydroindolones	Molindone*	10 mg

*Not licensed in the UK at time of going to press.

psychotic episode. The maintenance dosage of a conventional antipsychotic should be in the range of 300–600 CPZE/day.

A major problem in the maintenance treatment of a patient with schizophrenia is lack of adherence to the recommended pharmacological treatment regimen. The depot forms of conventional antipsychotics are particularly useful in this regard, because they can be administered once every 2–6 weeks and relieve the patient and caregiver of the burden of remembering to take medications daily. Depot preparations are used relatively frequently in the UK, but tend to be underused in the USA.

Adverse effects. Conventional antipsychotics have a broad range of adverse effects. The most important of these are extrapyramidal side effects (EPS), such as akinesia, dystonia and tremor. The side-effect profile of an antipsychotic is largely related to its potency or strength. High-potency antipsychotics (e.g. haloperidol, fluphenazine) are more likely to cause EPS, whereas low-potency antipsychotics (e.g. chlorpromazine, thioridazine) are more likely to cause sedation and orthostatic hypotension. EPS constitute a major cause of non-adherence to treatment. High-potency antipsychotics are also more likely to cause neuroleptic malignant syndrome (NMS), a syndrome characterized by muscle rigidity, autonomic instability (e.g. elevated pulse rate and blood pressure), fever and mental status changes. NMS is relatively rare (incidence of less than 1%) but, if left untreated, is associated with relatively high mortality.

The other major adverse effect associated with all conventional antipsychotics is tardive dyskinesia (TD). TD is characterized by abnormal, involuntary movements and primarily affects the muscles of the tongue and face. It may also involve the muscles of the extremities, pelvic girdle and/or diaphragm. TD varies in severity, with the majority of cases being relatively mild, but severe cases can be quite disabling and can lead to marked functional impairments. The cumulative incidence of conventional antipsychotic-induced TD is about 5% of patients per year of treatment.

Second-generation antipsychotics

The second-generation antipsychotics (Tables 9.2 and 9.3) were developed in an attempt to find effective antipsychotics with minimal potential for causing either EPS or TD. Unlike conventional

TABLE 9.2

Relative indications for the new and older antipsychotic drugs

Second-generation/atypical antipsychotics
- First- and second-line treatments
- Patients intolerant of conventional antipsychotic adverse effects, e.g. neurological or endocrinological
- Patients with refractory positive symptoms (clozapine)

Conventional antipsychotics
- Patients who are non-adherent: long-acting depot preparations
- During pregnancy
- Patients who fail to respond to second-generation antipsychotics
- If cost is a priority

TABLE 9.3

Second-generation antipsychotic drugs and their adverse effects

Drug	Main adverse effects	Comment
Clozapine	Agranulocytosis (reduced risk with regular monitoring) Sedation Seizures Salivation Weight gain Hyperlipidemias Diabetes mellitus	The only second-generation antipsychotic effective for refractory positive symptoms: clinical improvement in 30–60% Major risk factor for metabolic abnormalities
Risperidone	Insomnia, agitation EPS at higher doses Prolactin elevation	Evidence for enhanced relapse prevention Available in a long-acting intramuscular preparation
Olanzapine	Headache Sedation Weight gain Hyperlipidemias Diabetes mellitus	Few EPS Major risk factor for metabolic abnormalities
Quetiapine	Sedation Postural hypotension Dizziness Constipation	Few or no EPS Moderate risk factor for metabolic abnormalities
Amisulpride	Prolactin elevation EPS at higher doses	D_2 and D_3 specific
Ziprasidone*	Insomnia EPS at higher doses	Weight neutral Low risk factor for metabolic abnormalities
Aripiprazole	Mild dose-related EPS	Partial D_2 agonist Long half-life Low risk factor for metabolic abnormalities

*Not licensed in the UK at time of going to press.
EPS, extrapyramidal side effects.

antipsychotics, these agents are usually also potent $5HT_{2a}$ receptor antagonists. They may also have noradrenergic, histaminergic and cholinergic effects.

Clozapine. The first second-generation antipsychotic was clozapine. Although originally developed in the early 1960s, clozapine was not marketed in the UK and USA until 1990, because of concerns about the increased occurrence of agranulocytosis. In addition to its potent serotonergic $5HT_{2a}$ receptor antagonist activity, clozapine differs from conventional antipsychotics in its relative potency at the dopamine D_1 and D_4 receptors. Any one of these properties may be related to its superior efficacy for positive symptoms. Clozapine is the only second-generation antipsychotic that has been approved for the treatment of positive symptoms resistant to conventional antipsychotics (Case history 9.1). It is also effective for alleviating negative symptoms secondary to positive symptoms, EPS or dysphoric affect. Clozapine has not been shown to be effective for primary negative symptoms. Clozapine has been found to reduce suicidal ideation in schizophrenia.

Although clozapine causes few EPS and little TD, it does have a number of adverse effects that limit its use. The most serious of these is agranulocytosis, which occurs in up to 1% of treated patients, may be life-threatening and necessitates regular blood monitoring. However, the most clinically important adverse effects may be the substantial weight gain and disruptions of glucose and lipid metabolism that are associated with clozapine treatment. Clozapine has been shown to be responsible for the induction of new cases of type 2 diabetes mellitus. These drawbacks underscore the principle that all medications are associated with side effects and that the decreased occurrence of one serious set of adverse effects may be offset by the increased occurrence of an equally serious set of others. Other common clozapine-associated adverse effects include sedation, sialorrhea and seizures.

Other second-generation antipsychotics. The other second-generation antipsychotics share with clozapine potent $5\text{-}HT_{2a}$ antagonist properties, but differ in the degree to which they share the other pharmacological properties of clozapine. Several of the second-generation antipsychotics are known to cause substantial weight gain and disruption of glucose and lipid metabolism (see Table 9.3; Case history 9.2). They share with clozapine the reduced proclivity for causing EPS and TD. This latter property has led to their supplanting the conventional antipsychotics as first-line treatments for acute

---

Case history 9.1 – effective treatment of positive symptoms with clozapine

A 45-year-old white man had a 20-year history of paranoid schizophrenia. Despite treatment with adequate doses of both conventional (fluphenazine and haloperidol) and second-generation (risperidone and quetiapine) antipsychotics, he continued to exhibit persistent and severe positive symptoms.

The patient's symptoms included delusions that his neighbors were talking about him and that they broke into his house when he was not home. He also heard voices for several hours each day that commented on his behavior and told him to be on his guard.

The patient started treatment with clozapine at an initial dose of 25 mg, administered twice a day, and over the next 4 weeks the dose was increased to 400 mg/day. He experienced a modest decrease in symptoms, with decreased frequency in hearing voices, and he began to wonder if his concern about his neighbors was more related to his illness.

After 6 weeks, his dose was increased to 500 mg/day. The patient experienced a further reduction in his positive symptoms. The frequency of hearing voices decreased to one to two times per day for relatively short periods of time, and he began socializing with some of his neighbors, although these social interactions were still limited because of enduring suspiciousness.

His dose was increased to 600 mg/day, but no further improvement was noted. A blood sample was drawn, which showed that his plasma clozapine level was well above 350 ng/ml, the minimum therapeutic level. Therefore, no further changes to his medication regimen were made.

Fast Facts: Schizophrenia

Case history 9.2 – management of adverse metabolic effects with ziprasidone

A 24-year-old black woman presented to the clinic with a 9-month history of auditory hallucinations and the delusion that she had a special relationship with God, who spoke to her directly of his plans for the future of the world. She had no previous psychiatric history, although her family history included a diagnosis of bipolar disorder in her father.

The patient was obese and her mother was being treated with an oral hypoglycemic agent for type 2 diabetes mellitus. In light of her personal and family risk factors for diabetes mellitus, the patient began treatment with ziprasidone, 40 mg administered twice a day. In addition, her baseline fasting glucose level was measured, a lipid panel was obtained, and her weight, height and waist circumference were measured.

Her dose was increased to 80 mg, administered twice daily, and she had a moderate reduction in her symptoms. The fasting glucose and lipid panel measurements were repeated after 4 months of treatment and were found to remain in the normal range. She had gained a few pounds, but there was no notable change in her body mass index or waist circumference.

psychotic episodes and maintenance therapy. However, none of the other second-generation antipsychotics has yet been shown to be as effective as clozapine for treatment-resistant positive symptoms. Their putative efficacy for negative symptoms has not been sufficiently investigated to determine whether any of these new drugs are effective for both primary and secondary negative symptoms.

The Clinical Antipsychotic Trials of Intervention Effectiveness study

A major question that confronts clinicians is how to balance the relative efficacy and safety of conventional and second-generation antipsychotics. The Clinical Antipsychotic Trials of Intervention

Effectiveness (CATIE) study was designed to address this issue. The first phase of the study was an 18-month comparison of perphenazine (a conventional antipsychotic) with risperidone, olanzapine, quetiapine and ziprasidone (second-generation antipsychotics). The results were unexpected. First, 75% of the patients failed to complete the study on the medication to which they were randomly assigned. The median time to discontinuation was 6 months. Second, olanzapine was the most effective agent on the global measure of time to discontinuation. However, there were no efficacy differences among perphenazine and the other second-generation antipsychotics. Finally, olanzapine was found to be more likely to cause serious metabolic problems than were any of the other agents.

The CATIE study demonstrates the clinical principle that selection of the most appropriate antipsychotic treatment requires an individualized evaluation of the benefits and risks of a particular agent. The treatment history, medical history and medical risk factors must all be factored into the treatment decision. There is no single drug for every patient.

Treatment of negative symptoms

The treatment of negative symptoms is a major challenge facing clinicians. Conventional and second-generation antipsychotics are relatively effective for treating secondary negative symptoms, but leave untouched the primary avolitional syndrome described so eloquently by Kraepelin (see Chapter 1). The limited efficacy of antipsychotics has led to the investigation of alternative treatments for negative symptoms. Various approaches have been attempted based on specific neurochemical hypotheses of the pathophysiology of negative symptoms. One of the more promising strategies that has received some empirical support is the use of agents that increase the level of activity of the N-methyl-D-aspartate (NMDA) receptor. This approach is based on the proposition that negative symptoms are due to decreased glutamatergic activity. Glycine, D-serine and D-cycloserine all bind to the glycine site of the NMDA receptor and are required for NMDA receptor response to glutamate. In preliminary studies, they have been shown to be effective in ameliorating persistent negative symptoms. An alternative approach is to block the reuptake of glycine in the synaptic cleft. Initial studies with sarcosine suggest that this may also be an effective approach.

Treatment of cognitive impairments

Conventional antipsychotics have limited effects on the cognitive impairments of schizophrenia. They tend to produce small improvements across a broad range of cognitive functions, except for fine motor speed, which they worsen. Second-generation antipsychotics may have modest benefits for multiple cognitive processes, but it has not been established whether this represents a direct cognitive-enhancing effect or an indirect effect mediated through decreased adverse effects. Regardless, patients continue to exhibit pronounced cognitive impairments despite adequate treatment with the second-generation antipsychotic agents.

The limited benefit of antipsychotics has led to the search for alternative pharmacological mechanisms to enhance cognitive function. In this regard, cholinergic, dopaminergic, γ-aminobutyric acidergic and glutamatergic agents offer the most promise.

Treatment-resistant patients

Despite the advent of clozapine, a large percentage of patients continue to experience considerable residual positive symptoms. A number of agents have been used in combination with ongoing antipsychotic treatment in an attempt to alleviate these symptoms. The agents most commonly used in this regard are antiseizure medications (e.g. carbamazepine), antidepressants, benzodiazepines and lithium. However, although there are reports of small subgroups of patients who may benefit from combination therapy with one of these agents, there has not been a consistent demonstration of enhanced positive symptom efficacy when these drugs have been used in combination with antipsychotics. Rather, these drugs may be more effective when used to treat patients with persistent symptoms of anxiety, depression, hostility or mania.

Currently, the most common practice is to add a second antipsychotic medication in patients with residual positive symptoms. There is, however, little empirical evidence to support this practice.

Key points – pharmacological treatment

- The depot forms of conventional and second-generation antipsychotics are useful for patients who are non-adherent to their medications.
- Clozapine is the only second-generation antipsychotic that is effective for positive symptoms resistant to conventional antipsychotics.
- Second-generation antipsychotics other than clozapine have become the first-line treatments for acute psychotic episodes and maintenance therapy.
- Conventional and second-generation antipsychotics are relatively effective for treating secondary, but not primary, negative symptoms.
- Conventional antipsychotics have limited effects on the cognitive impairments of schizophrenia.
- Second-generation antipsychotics may have modest benefits for multiple cognitive processes.

Key references

Bilder RM, Goldman RS, Volavka J et al. Neurocognitive effects of clozapine, olanzapine, risperidone, and haloperidol in patients with chronic schizophrenia or schizoaffective disorder. *Am J Psychiatry* 2002;159:1018–28.

Buchanan RW, Breier A, Kirkpatrick B et al. Positive and negative symptom response to clozapine in schizophrenic patients with and without the deficit syndrome. *Am J Psychiatry* 1998;155:751–60.

Goff DC, Tsai G, Levitt J et al. A placebo-controlled trial of D-cycloserine added to conventional neuroleptics in patients with schizophrenia. *Arch Gen Psychiatry* 1999;56:21–7.

Green MF, Marder SR, Glynn SM et al. The neurocognitive effects of low-dose haloperidol: a two-year comparison with risperidone. *Biol Psychiatry* 2002;51:972–8.

Heresco-Levy U, Javitt DC, Ermilov M et al. Efficacy of high-dose glycine in the treatment of enduring negative symptoms of schizophrenia. *Arch Gen Psychiatry* 1999;56:29–36.

Kane J, Honigfeld G, Singer J, Meltzer H. Clozapine for the treatment-resistant schizophrenic: a double-blind comparison with chlorpromazine. *Arch Gen Psychiatry* 1988;45:789–96.

Keefe RS, Seidman LJ, Christensen BK et al. Comparative effect of atypical and conventional antipsychotic drugs on neuro-cognition in first-episode psychosis: a randomized, double-blind trial of olanzapine versus low doses of haloperidol. *Am J Psychiatry* 2004;161:985–95.

Lehman AF, Kreyenbuhl J, Buchanan RW et al. The Schizophrenia Patient Outcomes Research Team (PORT): updated treatment recommendations 2003. *Schizophr Bull* 2004;30:193–217.

Lieberman JA, Stroup TS, McEvoy JP et al. Effectiveness of antipsychotic drugs in patients with chronic schizophrenia. *N Engl J Med* 2005;353:1209–23.

Meltzer HY, Alphs L, Green AI et al. Clozapine treatment for suicidality in schizophrenia: International Suicide Prevention Trial (InterSePT). *Arch Gen Psychiatry* 2003;60:82–91.

Mishara AL, Goldberg TE. A meta-analysis and critical review of the effects of conventional neuroleptic treatment on cognition in schizophrenia: opening a closed book. *Biol Psychiatry* 2004;55:1013–22.

Rosenheck R, Tekell J, Peters J et al. Does participation in psychosocial treatment augment the benefit of clozapine? Department of Veterans Affairs Cooperative Study Group on Clozapine in Refractory Schizophrenia. *Arch Gen Psychiatry* 1998;55:618–25.

Tsai G, Lane HY, Yang P et al. Glycine transporter I inhibitor, N-methylglycine (sarcosine), added to antipsychotics for the treatment of schizophrenia. *Biol Psychiatry* 2004;55:452–6.

10 Psychosocial interventions and non-drug treatments

Psychosocial interventions have been a key part of the management of schizophrenia since the 1970s. At that time, the adverse impact of institutionalization on people with schizophrenia came to be realized, and this led to the increased development of community-based services. More recently, specific psychological techniques aimed at improving aspects of schizophrenia have also been evaluated (Table 10.1).

Modern service settings

Multidisciplinary teams are the core of community-based services for people with schizophrenia. These are effective when a case management model is used, so that one care coordinator develops and oversees the patient's entire care package. Different models of care management exist, but systematic reviews have shown that it is most effective when

TABLE 10.1

Effective psychological treatments in schizophrenia

Treatment	Strength of evidence base
Family intervention	++++
Cognitive therapy for persistent symptoms	+++
Cognitive therapy for acute symptoms	++
Cognitive therapy for relapse prevention	++
Cognitive therapy for prodromal symptoms	++
Social skills training	++
Motivational interventions in dual diagnosis	++
Cognitive remediation for chronic disabilities	++
Compliance therapy	+

++++, very strong; +++, strong; ++, moderate; +, unreplicated.

combined with assertive community treatment. This involves proactive community follow-up and delivery of as much care as possible in the home setting of the patient.

Getting patients back to work is also important. Systematic review has shown that supported employment programs, in which a patient is put into a real job and supported actively, outperform traditional sheltered employment approaches. Specialist rehabilitation services aim to reduce the enduring deficits in chronic schizophrenia and improve day-to-day social functioning.

Family interventions

The concept of high 'expressed emotion' within families as an environmental predictor of relapse in schizophrenia was suggested in the 1960s by Brown and Rutter. Families who showed overinvolvement or excessive criticism were associated with high relapse rates in schizophrenic individuals. Whether the high expressed emotion was the cause of the poor prognosis, or partly the effect of illness severity, has not been resolved. Nevertheless, family-based interventions aimed at enhancing coping strategies by education about the illness (Table 10.2) have been shown to improve prognosis.

A meta-analysis of the best randomized controlled trials, with a collective total of 350 patients and their families, found that such interventions, usually delivered over 9 months, were both effective and cost-effective. Patients who had family interventions showed lower relapse rates and improved drug compliance. Families valued the treatment and experienced less burden of care. This effect appears to be enduring and can be delivered to groups of families, with some evidence

TABLE 10.2

Components of an effective family intervention

- Engage families soon after acute admission
- Videos and seminars to educate the family about schizophrenia
- Early intervention in threatened relapse
- Teach problem-solving techniques

that this is the most cost-effective method. Family support combined with individual psychological techniques has been shown to reduce relapse rates in schizophrenia complicated by substance misuse.

Psychological treatment of positive symptoms

The idea that cognitive-behavioral treatments that are effective in major depression might be effective in treating positive psychotic symptoms is relatively new. Traditionally, these symptoms have been viewed, in the words of the phenomenologist Jaspers, as 'un-understandable'. This, coupled with the failure of psychoanalytical treatments for schizophrenia in the 1950s and 1960s, left a legacy of skepticism about psychological approaches.

Since the mid-1990s, trials have shown that cognitive-behavioral therapy (CBT) can be effective for persistent psychotic symptoms in chronic schizophrenia when given in addition to routine care. The effect size in four large, independent, randomized controlled trials is about the same as that for clozapine.

Components of this technique are shown in Table 10.3. Which of these components is the most important remains to be clarified.

TABLE 10.3

Components of cognitive-behavioral therapy in schizophrenia

Cognitive components
- Identifying links between thoughts, emotions and behaviors
- Identifying automatic thoughts
- Hypothesis testing about abnormal beliefs; reframing attributions
- Identifying and enhancing coping strategies

Behavioral elements
- Symptom monitoring; use of diary
- Distraction techniques; focusing strategies for 'voices'
- Graded task assignment
- Anxiety management and relaxation techniques

Recent trials have also shown that these techniques, added to drug treatment, may improve outcomes for psychotic symptoms in acute psychosis, including first-episode schizophrenia.

Relapse prevention

The mainstay of relapse prevention in schizophrenia is maintenance drug treatment. Relapse risk can be reduced by 50% with added CBT if early signs of relapse, such as racing thoughts or suspiciousness, appear (Case history 10.1).

Patients with substance use in addition to psychosis ('dual diagnosis') are especially prone to relapse. A combination of CBT and so-called motivational interviewing, a strategy successful in uncomplicated substance use, can reduce relapse rates. In motivational

---

Case history 10.1 – cognitive-behavioral therapy helps to reduce persecutory delusions

A 40-year-old man had a 15-year history of schizophrenia, which comprised a persistent systemized set of persecutory delusions that affected how he behaved. He avoided going out into the street as he believed that passersby stared at him, which upset him.

These symptoms failed to improve substantially with second-generation antipsychotic drugs, including clozapine. Cognitive-behavioral assessment revealed his most preoccupying symptom to be the delusion of reference that passersby stared at him, about which he admitted to being 99% certain.

The patient was led through a behavioral experiment in which he walked down the street wearing a bright green bow tie, so that he could judge how it felt when people genuinely stared at him. He was then asked to consider a range of alternative explanations, such as fatigue, for why his beliefs arose.

After ten twice-weekly sessions, his beliefs were less strongly held and less distressing, and he was able to venture out alone.

interviewing, patients are helped to review what they have to gain or lose by not accepting treatment and remaining or becoming ill. The clinician helps patients to generate a series of possible options, of which taking drug treatment is one, and to look at the consequences of each decision.

Improving adherence to medication

Poor compliance with, or adherence to, drug treatment is not unique to schizophrenia. Reasons for non-adherence to antipsychotic drugs are given in Table 10.4.

Psychological approaches can improve adherence to medication. Education and explanation about the precise benefits and risks of drug treatment in individual cases should be the starting point, establishing a collaborative approach. Motivational interviewing has been shown to reduce relapse through increased medication adherence.

Cognitive remediation

Neuropsychological impairments have been shown to be strong predictors of outcome. Cognitive remediation in chronic schizophrenia aims to train patients on specific neuropsychological tasks. Recent trials have shown this to be effective and that the gains may generalize into wider aspects of social functioning.

TABLE 10.4

Contributors to antipsychotic drug non-adherence

- Adverse effects, particularly extrapyramidal side effects, weight gain and sexual dysfunction
- Perceived lack of efficacy
- Inadequate information
- Complex prescribing regimens
- Stigma
- Delusional beliefs
- Lack of insight

Key points – psychosocial interventions and non-drug treatments

- Family interventions are known to be effective in reducing relapse.
- Cognitive-behavioral therapy (CBT) in addition to drug treatment reduces persistent positive symptoms. CBT can also abort relapses if targeted at early signs.
- Motivational intervention techniques can reduce street drug use and enhance treatment compliance.
- Cognitive remediation reduces some cognitive deficits in chronic schizophrenia.

Key references

Barrowclough C, Haddock G, Tarrier N et al. Randomised controlled trial of motivational interviewing, cognitive behavior therapy, and family intervention for patients with comorbid schizophrenia and substance use disorders. *Am J Psychiatry* 2001;158:1706–13.

Gumley A, O'Grady M, McNay L et al. Early intervention for relapse in schizophrenia: results of a 12-month randomized controlled trial of cognitive behavioural therapy. *Psychol Med* 2003;33:419–31.

McFarlane WR, Lukens E, Link B et al. Multiple-family groups and psychoeducation in the treatment of schizophrenia. *Arch Gen Psychiatry* 1995;52:679–87.

Meuser KT, Berenbaum H. Psychodynamic treatment of schizophrenia: is there a future? *Psychol Med* 1990;20:253–62.

Tarrier N, Barrowclough C, Porceddu K, Fitzpatrick E. The Salford family intervention project: relapse rates of schizophrenia at five and eight years. *Br J Psychiatry* 1994;165:829–32.

Tarrier N, Lewis S, Haddock G et al. Cognitive-behavioural therapy in first-episode and early schizophrenia. 18-month follow-up of a randomised controlled trial. *Br J Psychiatry* 2004;184:231–9.

Tarrier N, Wykes T. Is there evidence that cognitive behaviour therapy is an effective treatment for schizophrenia? A cautious or cautionary tale? *Behav Res Ther* 2004;42:1377–401.

First episodes of schizophrenia often go undetected and untreated for long periods of time. The median duration of positive psychotic symptoms before detection is 12–24 weeks, but in many cases symptoms endure for much longer before detection, particularly if negative symptoms are taken into account. The duration of untreated psychosis (DUP) is strongly associated with response to treatment and speed to remission in the first episode, although it is still disputed whether this is truly a causal link. Nonetheless, this observation is the main impetus behind the increasing focus on early detection and treatment of the first episode of schizophrenia.

Early detection

There are two linked questions. First, is it possible to detect, and so treat, people earlier in their first episode? Second, if so, will earlier treatment lead to better outcomes?

The answer to the first question is almost certainly yes. Some of the reasons for delayed detection are given in Table 11.1. Public education, training of family physicians and youth workers in recognizing early signs, and specialist rapid assessment teams have been shown in pilot early-intervention services to reduce median DUP to 6 weeks, with a concomitant reduction in symptom severity by the time of treatment initiation.

TABLE 11.1

Reasons for long duration of untreated psychosis

- Underrecognition of psychotic symptoms
- Delayed referral to specialist services
- Normal variation in individual health beliefs
- Specific symptoms: social withdrawal, loss of insight
- Ineffective first treatments

It is likely that earlier treatments lead to a better outcome, but this is technically still unproven. Randomized controlled trials of whole services are being attempted. Only part of the link between long DUP and poor outcome is explained by the fact that a long DUP leads to more severe symptoms by the time treatment is commenced (Table 11.2). One recently highlighted caveat is that impaired premorbid function, known by itself to predict poor outcome, may also lead to long DUP.

Optimal treatment in the first episode

Key elements of an early-intervention strategy are given in Table 11.3. Outcome from the first episode is good in 85% of cases, with remission usually achieved within 3 months.

Patients in the first episode are responsive to relatively low doses of antipsychotic drugs, and treatment should be started with the equivalent of haloperidol, 2 mg daily or less. Similarly, first-episode patients are sensitive to the adverse effects of drugs, and the second-generation antipsychotics are to be preferred.

Although remission from the first episode is not difficult to achieve, 50% of cases will relapse over the next 2 years and 80% over the next 5 years. With each relapse, about one in six will not subsequently achieve remission.

TABLE 11.2

Possible reasons for link between long duration of DUP and poor outcome

- More severe symptoms by the time treatment is started
- Active psychosis is neurotoxic through dopaminergic or glutamatergic processes
- Prolonged psychosis causes progressive loss of social frameworks (e.g. job, family)
- Long DUP and poor outcome both result from a third variable (e.g. poor premorbid function)

DUP, duration of untreated psychosis.

TABLE 11.3

Key elements of an early-intervention service

- Rapid response and assessment
- Youth-friendly and non-stigmatizing
- Family and caregiver education and support
- Effective psychological treatments
- Second-generation antipsychotic drug treatments
- Assertive treatment of refractory symptoms

Prodromal states: can schizophrenia be prevented?

It is possible to identify in the community individuals who are at very high risk of developing schizophrenia in the near future. Table 11.4 summarizes the descriptions of such cases with so-called prodromal or ultra-high-risk symptoms.

Overall, follow-up studies of individuals seeking help for these symptoms show that 20–40% will develop schizophrenia or a related psychotic disorder over the next 12 months. Given effective drug or psychological interventions at this prodromal stage, it may be feasible to prevent, delay or at least ameliorate subsequent psychosis in such cases (Case history 11.1). Randomized trials have shown that both second-generation antipsychotic drug treatments and cognitive therapy reduce rates of transition to schizophrenia.

TABLE 11.4

Operational definitions of at-risk prodromal states

- First-degree family history of psychosis plus recent functional deterioration
- Schizotypal personality plus recent functional deterioration
- Brief, limited, intermittent (less than 1 week) psychotic symptoms
- Attenuated (below diagnostic threshold) psychotic symptoms

Adapted from Yung et al. 1996.

The ethical issues relating to the treatment of individuals, most of whom will not go on in any case to develop psychosis, still need to be fully explored, but this is one of today's most promising research areas.

Case history 11.1 – early intervention for attenuated psychotic symptoms

A 19-year-old student who had been using increasing amounts of cannabis had, for the past 3 months, developed the unpleasant impression that people might have been talking about him behind his back, and on two occasions he heard what he thought could have been whispered comments about him. He was distressed about this and consulted student health services.

At the interview, he was anxious but not markedly depressed. He had ideas of reference but recognized that these were likely to be due to his imagination, as were the perceived whisperings. The patient did not meet any diagnostic criteria for a full psychotic disorder. It was explained to him that he had attenuated psychotic symptoms that might deteriorate.

The patient agreed to a program of cognitive therapy with the opportunity of low-dose antipsychotic drug treatment if his symptoms failed to improve. He remained well a year later.

Key points – early intervention

- Duration of untreated psychosis is usually 3–6 months.
- The longer the delay in treatment the worse the clinical outcome.
- Early detection has been shown to be possible.
- Second-generation drugs are preferred.
- Treatment of prodromal cases with cognitive-behavioral or drug therapy may prevent or delay schizophrenia.

Key references

Drake RJ, Haley CJ, Akhtar S, Lewis SW. Causes and consequences of duration of untreated psychosis in schizophrenia. *Br J Psychiatry* 2000;177:511–5.

Haddock G, Lewis S. Psychological interventions in early psychosis. *Schizophr Bull* 2005;31:697–704.

Klosterkotter J, Hellmich M, Steinmeyer EM, Schultze-Lutter F. Diagnosing schizophrenia in the initial prodromal phase. *Arch Gen Psychiatry* 2001;58:158–64.

Marshall M, Lewis S, Lockwood A et al. Association between duration of untreated psychosis and outcome in cohorts of first-episode patients: a systematic review. *Arch Gen Psychiatry* 2005;62:975–83.

McGlashan TH, Zipursky RB, Perkins D et al. Randomized, double-blind trial of olanzapine versus placebo in patients prodromally symptomatic for psychosis. *Am J Psychiatry* 2006;163:790–9.

McGorry PD, Yung AR, Phillips LJ et al. Randomized controlled trial of interventions designed to reduce the risk of progression to first-episode psychosis in a clinical sample with subthreshold symptoms. *Arch Gen Psychiatry* 2002;59:921–8.

Morrison AP, French P, Walford L et al. Cognitive therapy for the prevention of psychosis in people at ultra-high risk: randomised controlled trial. *Br J Psychiatry* 2004;185:291–7.

Yung AR, McGorry PD, McFarlane CA et al. Monitoring and care of young people at incipient risk of psychosis. *Schizophr Bull* 1996;22:283–303.

Useful addresses

UK

British Association for Behavioural and Cognitive Psychotherapies
The Globe Centre, PO Box 9
Accrington BB5 0XB
Tel: +44 (0)1254 875277
babcp@babcp.com
www.babcp.org.uk

British Association for Counselling and Psychotherapy
BACP House
15 St John's Business Park
Lutterworth LE17 4HB
Tel: 0870 443 5252
bacp@bacp.co.uk
www.bacp.co.uk

British Association for Psychopharmacology
BAP Office, 36 Cambridge Place
Hills Road, Cambridge CB2 1NS
Tel: +44 (0)1223 358395
www.bap.org.uk

The British Psychological Society
St Andrews House
48 Princess Road East
Leicester LE1 7DR
Tel: +44 (0)116 254 9568
enquiry@bps.org.uk
www.bps.org.uk

Making Space
(Helps people with schizophrenia and other mental illnesses cope more effectively)
46 Allen Street, Warrington
Cheshire WA2 7JB
Tel: +44 (0)1925 571680
www.makingspace.co.uk

Mental Health Alliance
c/o The Sainsbury Centre for Mental Health, 134–138 Borough High St
London SE1 1LB
www.mentalhealthalliance.org.uk

Mental Health Foundation
9th Floor, Sea Containers House
20 Upper Ground, London SE1 9QB
Tel: +44 (0)20 7803 1101
mhf@mhf.org.uk
www.mhf.org.uk

Mind (The Mental Health Charity)
15–19 Broadway
London E15 4BQ
Tel: +44 (0)20 8519 2122
Mind*info*Line: 0845 766 0163
(Mon–Fri 9.15 AM–5.15 PM)
contact@mind.org.uk
www.mind.org.uk

National Electronic Library for Mental Health
www.library.nhs.uk/mentalhealth

Rethink (formerly the National Schizophrenia Fellowship)
Head Office, 5th Floor
Royal London House
22–25 Finsbury Square
London EC2A 1DX
Tel: 0845 456 0455
Helpline: +44 (0)20 8974 6814
(Mon–Fri 10 AM–3 PM)
info@rethink.org
www.rethink.org

The Royal College of Psychiatrists
17 Belgrave Square
London SW1X 8PG
Tel: +44 (0)20 7235 2351
rcpsych@rcpsych.ac.uk
www.rcpsych.ac.uk

SAMH (Scottish Association for Mental Health)
Cumbrae House, 15 Carlton Court
Glasgow G5 9JP
Tel: +44 (0)141 568 7000
enquire@samh.org.uk
www.samh.org.uk

SANE & SANELINE
1st Floor, Cityside House
40 Adler Street, London E1 1EE
Tel: +44 (0)20 7375 1002
SANELINE: 0845 767 8000
(1 PM–11 PM every day)
info@sane.org.uk
www.sane.org.uk

UK Mental Health Research Network
PO Box 77, Institute of Psychiatry
Kings College London
De Crespigny Park, London SE5 8AF
Tel: +44 (0)20 7848 0699
mhrn@iop.kcl.ac.uk
www.mhrn.info

USA
American Academy of Child and Adolescent Psychiatry
3615 Wisconsin Avenue, NW
Washington, DC 20016-3007
Tel: +1 202 966 7300
clinical@aacap.org (clinical practice)
www.aacap.org

American College of Neuropsychopharmacology
545 Mainstream Drive, Suite 110
Nashville, TN 37228
Tel: +1 615 324 2360
acnp@acnp.org
www.acnp.org

American Psychiatric Association
1000 Wilson Blvd, Suite 1825
Arlington, VA 22209-3901
Tel: +1 703 907 7300
apa@psych.org
www.psych.org

American Psychiatric Nurses
Association
1555 Wilson Boulevard
Suite 602, Arlington, VA 22209
Toll-free: 1 866 243 2443
www.apna.org

American Psychological
Association
750 First Street, NE
Washington, DC 20002-4242
Tel: +1 202 336 5500
Toll-free: 1 800 374 2721
www.apa.org

American Psychotherapy
Association
2750 E Sunshine Street
Springfield, MO 65804
Toll-free: 1 800 205 9165
www.americanpsychotherapy.com

Center for Psychiatric
Rehabilitation
940 Commonwealth Avenue, West
Boston, MA 02215
Tel: +1 617 353 3549
www.bu.edu/cpr

Mental Health America
(formerly the National Mental
Health Associaton)
2000 N Beauregard Street
6th Floor, Alexandria, VA 22311
Tel: +1 703 684 7722
Toll-free: 1 800 969 6642
www.nmha.org

NARSAD: The Mental Health
Research Association
(formerly the National Alliance
for Research on Schizophrenia
and Depression)
60 Cutter Mill Road, Suite 404
Great Neck, NY 11021
Tel: +1 516 829 0091
Helpline: 1 800 829 8289
info@narsad.org
www.narsad.org

National Alliance on Mental Illness
Colonial Place Three
2107 Wilson Blvd, Suite 300
Arlington, VA 22201-3042
Tel: +1 703 524 7600
Helpline: 1 800 950 6264
www.nami.org

National Institute of Mental
Health
6001 Executive Boulevard
Room 8184, MSC 9663
Bethesda, MD 20892-9663
Tel: +1 301 443 4513
Toll-free: 1 866 615 6464
nimhinfo@nih.gov
www.nimh.nih.gov

SAMHSA's National Mental
Health Information Center
PO Box 42557
Washington, DC 20015
Tel: +1 240 747 5484
Toll-free: 1 800 789 2647
(Mon–Fri 8.30 AM–12 noon)
www.mentalhealth.samhsa.gov

Society of Biological Psychiatry
c/o Mayo Clinic Jacksonville
Research – Birdsall 310
4500 San Pablo Road
Jacksonville, FL 32224
Tel: +1 904 953 2842
www.sobp.org

Society for Neuroscience
1121 14th Street, NW, Suite 1010
Washington, DC 20005
Tel: +1 202 962 4000
info@sfn.org
apu.sfn.org

International
Association of European
Psychiatrists
5, quai de Paris
67000 Strasbourg, France
Tel: +33 (0)3 88 23 99 30
aep.strasbourg@wanadoo.fr
www.aep.lu

Collegium Internationale
Neuro-Psychopharmacologicum
CINP Central Office
1 Tennant Avenue
College Milton South, E Kilbride
Glasgow G74 5NA, UK
Tel: +44 (0)1355 244930
www.cinp.org

European College of
Neuropsychopharmacology
ECNP-Office, PO Box 85410
3508 AK Utrecht, The Netherlands
Tel: +31 (0)30 253 8567
secretariat@ecnp.nl
www.ecnp.eu

European Federation of
Psychologists' Associations
EFPA Head Office
Grasmarkt 105/18
B-1000 Brussels, Belgium
Tel: +32 (0)2 503 49 53
www.efpa.be

Global Alliance of Mental Illness Advocacy Networks
GAMIAN, 308 Seaview Avenue
Staten Island, NY 10305, USA
Tel: +1 718 351 1717
www.gamian.org

International Brain Research Organization
255 rue Saint Honoré
75001 Paris, France
Tel: +33 (0)1 46 47 92 92
admin@ibro.info
www.ibro.org

International Early Psychosis Association
IEPA Locked Bag 10, Parkville
Victoria 3052, Australia
Tel: +61 (3) 9342 2837
info@iepa.org.au
www.iepa.org.au

World Federation of Societies of Biological Psychiatry
Zum Ehrenshain 34
22885 Barsbüttel, Germany
Tel: +49 (0)4067 088290
info@wfsbp.org
www.wfsbp.org

World Psychiatric Association
WPA Secretariat
Psychiatric Hospital
2, ch. du Petit-Bel-Air
1225 Chêne-Bourg, Switzerland
Tel: +41 (0)22 305 5730
wpasecretariat@wpanet.org
www.wpanet.org

Index

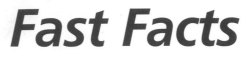
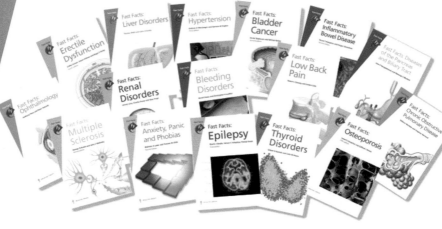